DIAGNOSTICS OF TRADITIONAL CHINESE MEDICINE

Compiled by   Shao Nian Fang
Translated by   Wang Qi Liang
Examined and
Revised by   Wang Qi Liang

Shandong Science and Technology
Press, 1990

First Edition 1990

Published by SHANDONG SCIENCE AND
TECHNOLOGY PRESS
Yu Han Lu, Jinan, China
Printed by WEIFANG XINHUA PRINTING HOUSE
99 Gongnong Road, Weifang, China
DISTRIBUTED BY CHINA INTERNATIONAL BOOK
TRADING CORPORATION
21 CHEGONGZHUANG XILU, BEIJING, CHINA
P. O. BOX 399, BEIJING, CHINA
POSTAL ZONE: 100044

Printed in the People's Republic of China

PREFACE

Diagnostics is an intermediate branch of learning which links preclinical medicine and clinical medicine. It is a prerequisite for the choice of therapeutic measures. Obviously, without a clear and definite diagnosis, there will be an erroneous treatment.

In this book, elementary knowledge about diagnostics of Traditional Chinese Medicine is introduced; Four Kinds of Diagnostic Examination, Eight Principal Syndromes, and Differentiation of Symptoms and Signs according to various theoretical systems are discussed in a pithy style. To make them easy to understand, selected Medical Reports written by well-known doctors are included.

We hope this book will be of some use to those who are interested in Traditional Chinese Medicine.

Compiler
1989. 4

CONTENTS

Chapter I Introduction ··· 1

Chapter II Four Kinds of Diagnostic Examination ·· 3

  Section 1. Inspection ··· 3
    I. Inspection of expression, vitality, and mental state ······························ 3
    II. Inspection of complexion ·· 3
    III. Inspection of configuration, posture, deportment, and movement ········· 5
    IV. Inspection of the tongue ··· 6
    V. Inspection of the head, neck, Five Sense Organs, and Lower Apertures ··· 16
    VI. Inspection of the skin ··· 24
    VII. Inspection of Superficial Venules of the Index Finger ······················· 26
    VIII. Inspection of various discharge ··· 28

  Section 2. Auscultation and smelling ·· 29
    I. Auscultation ·· 29
    II. Smelling ··· 34

  Section 3. Interrogation ·· 35
    I. Cold and heat ·· 36
    II. Perspiration ·· 38
    III. The head and body ·· 39
    IV. The chest, hypochondria, epigastrium, and abdomen ························ 43
    V. The ear and the eye ·· 45
    VI. Diet and taste ··· 47
    VII. Sleep ··· 49
    VIII. Defecation and urination ··· 50
    IX. Menstruation, leucorrhea, pregnancy, and child-bearing ···················· 52
    X. Children ·· 56
    XI. Anamnesis ··· 57
    XII. Family history ··· 58
    XIII. Life style ··· 58

  Section 4. Pulse feeling and palpation ·· 58
    I. Pulse feeling ··· 58
    II. Palpation ··· 67

Chapter III Syndrome Differentiation ·· 68

  Section 1. Differentiation of Eight Principal Syndromes ··························· 68
    I. Exterior and Interior ··· 69
    II. Cold and Heat ·· 71

  III. Asthenia and Sthenia ··· 75
  IV. Yin and Yang ··· 78
  V. Complicated states of Eight Principal Syndromes ··· 79
  Annex Illustrative Medical Reports (Abridged) ··· 80
Section 2. Differentiation of Visceral syndrome ··· 82
  I. Differentiation of Heart syndrome ··· 82
  II. Differentiation of Small Intestine syndrome ··· 84
  III. Differentiation of Spleen syndrome ··· 84
  IV. Differentiation of Stomach syndrome ··· 86
  V. Differentiation of Lung syndrome ··· 87
  VI. Differentiation of Large Intestine syndrome ··· 88
  VII. Differentiation of Kidney syndrome ··· 89
  VIII. Differentiation of Urinary Bladder syndrome ··· 90
  IX. Differentiation of Liver syndrome ··· 90
  X. Differentiation of Gallbladder syndrome ··· 93
  XI. Differentiation of Pericardium syndrome ··· 93
  XII. Differentiation of Triple Energizer syndrome ··· 94
  XIII. Complicated syndromes of Parenchymatous Viscera ··· 94
  Annex Illustrative Medical Reports (Abridged) ··· 95
Section 3. Differentiation of syndromes of Vital Energy, Blood, and Fluid ··· 98
  I. Differentiation of Vital Energy syndrome ··· 98
  II. Differentiation of Blood syndrome ··· 99
  III. Complicated manifestations of Vital Energy and Blood syndrome ··· 100
  IV. Differentiation of Fluid syndrome ··· 100
  Annex Illustrative Medical Reports (Abridged) ··· 101
Section 4. Differentiation of Meridian syndrome ··· 103
Section 5. Differentiation of Exogenous Febrile Disease according
    to the theory of Six Meridians ··· 104
  I. Taiyang syndrome ··· 104
  II. Yangming syndrome ··· 104
  III. Shaoyang syndrome ··· 105
  IV. Taiyin syndrome ··· 105
  V. Shaoyin syndrome ··· 105
  VI. Jueyin syndrome ··· 105
Section 6. Differentiation of syndromes of Epidemic Febrile Disease ··· 106
  I. Theory of Defence-Energy-Nutrient-Blood Systems ··· 106
  II. Theory of Triple Energizer ··· 107
  III. Identification of Epidemic Febrile Diseases ··· 108
  Annex Illustrative Medical Reports (Abridged) ··· 108
References ··· 112

CHAPTER I   INTRODUCTION

Diagnostics deals with the method for examining disease conditions, the differentiation of symptoms and signs, and the identification of pathogenesis and causes of disease, thereby to find out a proper treatment. In Traditional Chinese Medicine, these are carried out in line with different theoretical systems from those of Western Medicine. As to details of the rationale of TCM, such as theories of Yin-Yang, Five Elements, Outward Manifestations of Viscera, Meridians and Collaterals, etc., please refer to relevant expoundings in classics of TCM.

Features of Diagnostics of TCM

I. *The concept of wholism*

TCM holds that there is a correspondence between mankind and the universe. The structure, physiological functions, and pathological changes of the human body may be regarded as a microcosm; while those of the natural environment a macrocosm. Ordinary changes of climates are beneficial to our health, extraordinary changes may be causes of disease.

II. *The integrity of human body*

Through Meridians, Collaterals, Tendons, and the circulation of Vital Energy and Blood, various parts of the body are linked together as an unity. Thus, a local pathologic process may influence the whole body, a general pathogenic process may manifest itself firstly at a local part. Disorders of the upper part may be transmitted to the lower part, disorders of the lower part may be transmitted to the upper part. Mental changes may impair the function of internal organs, dysfunction of internal organs may influence the mental state. It goes without saying that any pathologic change within the body has to manifest itself outwardly, and may be detected by meticulous and comprehensive examination.

III. *Four kinds of diagnostic examination*

Four Kinds of Diagnostic Examination in TCM consist of inspection, auscultation and olfaction, interrogation, and pulse feeling and palpation. Among them, inspection of the tongue and its coating and pulse feeling are characteristics of TCM diagnostics.

IV. *Unique ideology and methodology in syndrome differentiation*

In TCM, symptoms and signs are analysed and synthesized according to theories of Eight Principles, Six Meridians, Outward Manifestations of Viscera, and Defence-Energy-Nutrient-Blood Systems, etc. All these theories are based on rich clinical experiences, established and developed by numerous well-known doctors from generation to generation, and proved to be useful up to now.

V. *Causes of disease*

According to TCM, causes of disease are classified as endopathic factors (or Seven Emotions: joy, anger, melancholy, anxiety, grief, fear, and terror); exopathic factors (Extraordinary Six Climatic Conditions: Wind, Cold, Summer-Heat, Wetness, Dryness, and Fire); and non-exo-nonendopathic factors, such as improper diets, trauma, bites by beasts or insects, etc.

CHAPTER II FOUR KINDS OF DIAGNOSTIC EXAMINATION

Section 1.   Inspection

I. *Inspection of expression, vitality, and mental state*

Through inspection of expression, vitality, and mental state which are reflected prominently in the lustre and movement of one's eyes, we may assess the vicissitude of his (her) Essence and Vital Energy, and the degree of seriousness of the disease.

1. Bright eyes signify an exuberant state of Essence and Vital Energy, or the Healthy Energy has not been impaired, or the disease is not serious and easy to be cured.

2. Listless eyes with stupid pupils signify the depletion or exhaustion of Essence and Vital Energy, or the Healthy Energy has been greatly impaired, or a seriously ill condition.

3. Pseudo vitality occurs in extremely weakened patients who have been suffered from protracted serious illness. Such patients may suddenly take a turn for the "better". Their eyes become bright, or they may become talkative, hyperorexia, etc. This is the so-called "a flash of lucidity of the dying", or the momentary recovery of consciousness just before death.

4. Abnormal expression, vitality, or mental state may be seen in patients suffering from depressive psychosis (apathy, dementia, etc.), mania (dysphoria, bellicosity, etc.), or epilepsy (sudden faint, tic of limbs, etc.).

II. *Inspection of complexion (lustre and colour)*

1. Normal complexion varies with races, living and working conditions, seasons, etc. Drinking of alcoholic liquor, emotional excitement, or intense labour may also influence one's complexion, but

these should not be mistaken as manifestations of disease.

2. Abnormal complexion

1) White: Generally, white or pale complexion implies Asthenia or a cold syndrome. It may also occur in a collapse due to massive hemorrhage, or a syncope due to the exhaustion of Vital Energy.

White or glossy white generally signifies the deficiency of Yang or Vital Energy. Pale or fading yellow generally signifies the deficiency of Blood. Sudden pale with dripping cold sweat generally signifies the collapse of Yang or Vital Energy.

2) Yellow: Yellow complexion generally implies Wetness-Heat, or Asthenia. Bright yellow complexion all over the body with yellow sclera or Yang jaundice is caused by Wetness-Heat. Dim yellow complexion all over the body with yellow sclera or Yin jaundice is caused by Wetness-Cold.

In tympanites, there are sallow complexion and varicose on the abdominal wall.

3) Red: Generally, red complexion implies a heat syndrome. Flushing may be caused by exopathic fever or internal heat. Redness at both zygomatic regions usually signifies the flaring of Fire caused by Yin deficiency. Tender redness wandering on a pale face is a sign of "Floating Yang" which indicates a pseudo heat syndrome in the upper part of the body and a genuine cold syndrome in the lower part of the body.

4) Blue: Generally, blue complexion implies Wind, Cold, or pain. Blue colour appearing at the locale between eyebrows, the bridge of the nose, or the perioral region generally signifies infantile convulsion. Cyanotic complexion and lips generally signify the deficiency of Heart Yang. Bluish black complexion generally signifies an extreme interior Cold, or serious pain in the abdomen.

5) Black: Black complexion generally implies Cold, pain, or Kidney Asthenia. Yellowish black complexion may be seen in jaundice due to sexual indulgence or immoderate drinking of alcoholic liquor.

3. Ten essentials in inspection of complexion

In Qing Dynasty, Wang Hong had proposed that ten essentials

should be discriminated carefully.

1) Shallow or hidden: A shallow complexion indicates an exterior syndrome, a hidden complexion indicates an interior syndrome.

2) Lucid or turbid: A lucid complexion indicates an Yang syndrome, a turbid complexion indicates an Yin syndrome.

3) Light or dense: A light complexion indicates Asthenia of Healthy Energy, a dense complexion indicates Sthenia of pathogenic evil.

4) Diffused or stagnated: A diffused complexion indicates a new disease or a disease is going to be relieved, a stagnated complexion indicates a protracted disease or the pathogenic evil accumulates gradually.

5) Fresh or withered: A fresh complexion indicates a chance of survival, a withered complexion indicates the coming of death.

When the former changes into the latter, or vice versa, there will be corresponding change of location, nature, or prognosis of the disease.

III. *Inspection of configuration, posture, deportment, and movement*

1. Configuration

Obese people are generally deficient in Yang and Vital Energy, excessive in wetness and Phlegm. They are apt to suffer from apoplexy.

Lean people are generally deficient in Yin or Essence. They are apt to suffer from asthenic Fire.

When a patient is bedridden and extremely emaciated with deep sunken socket of eyeballs, it signifies a critical condition.

2. Posture and deportment

Dysphoria, restlessness, lifting one's quilt or taking off one's clothes, facing outwardly are signs of a heat, Yang syndrome.

Lying still in bed, desire for additional or thick quilt, facing inwardly are signs of a cold, Yin syndrome.

Lying in bed, inability of sitting up because of dizziness or vertigo are generally due to the deficiency of Vital Energy and Blood.

Sitting and facing upward, dyspnea with retention of phlegm in the air passage are generally due to Lung Sthenia.

Sitting with one's head drooping, shortness of breath, and disinclination to talk are generally due to Lung Asthenia.

Orthopnea, cough, inability of lying in bed, usually having a relapse in winter signify a recurrent Fluid retention syndrome.

Orthopnea, dropsy, and palpitation are generally due to the Asthenia of Heart-Kidney Yang.

Moreover, drooping head with sunken and lustreless eyes are signs of the exhaustion of Vitality. Crooked back with drooping shoulders signifies the exhaustion of Visceral Energy within the chest. Aching of the waist which cannot be turned are often due to Kidney Asthenia.

Floccitation is a sign of dying.

3. Movement

Opisthotonus and tic of limbs are manifestations of endogenous stirring of Liver Wind or the stirring of Wind due to exuberant Heart. These are often seen in infantile convulsion, epilepsy, tetanus, etc.

Twitching of the lip, cheek, eyelids, or digits now and then are manifestations of malnourishment of Tendons and Vessels due to Blood Asthenia, or they are omens of Wind stirring.

Weakness of arms and legs without pain signifies a syndrome of flaccidity.

Arthralgia is generally caused by Wind-Cold-Wetness.

Hemiplegia, deviation of the eye and mouth, stiff tongue, dysphasia are manifestation of apoplexy. Apoplexy with sudden onset of faint or loss of consciousness implies internal organs are involved. Apoplexy with a sober mind implies only Meridians and/or Collaterals are attacked, or it is the sequelae of a stroke which had attacked internal organs.

IV. *Inspection of the tongue*

This is a special domain of diagnostic examination in Traditional Chinese Medicine, which includes the inspection of both the tongue proper and its coating.

1. Rationale

1) The tongue is the opening of Heart, which is the chief of all

internal organs.

2) The tongue is connected with Kidney, Spleen, and Liver according to the Theory of Meridians; besides, Governor Vessel Meridian links up with the tongue.

3) The coating of the tongue is an outward exhibition of Stomach Energy.

2. Distribution of internal organs on lingual surface

There are two viewpoints regarding the distribution of internal organs on lingual surface:

1) The tip of the tongue corresponds to the upper part of Stomach; the middle part of the tongue corresponds to the middle part of Stomach; the root of the tongue corresponds to the lower part of Stomach.

2) The root of the tongue belongs to Kidney; the middle part or the whole surface of the tongue belongs to Stomach; the tip of the tongue belongs to Heart; the lateral sides of the tongue belong to Liver-Gallbladder; four boundaries of the tongue belong to Spleen.

3. Method of inspection and matters needing attention

The proper method is as follows: Let the patient sit upright facing natural light source, open his (her) mouth to the utmost, stretch the tongue out of his (her) mouth freely with its tip pointing slightly downward to expose the whole body of the tongue.

Diets and drugs may influence the colour and appearance of lingual coating. For example, milk may dye the coating in white; Coptis Chinensis powder, loquat, riboflavin may dye the coating in yellow; olive, sour plums, pills made of Chinese Medical Herbs, etc., may dye the coating in black; dregs of peanuts, melon seeds, and bean products, which are rich in fats, may adhere to the lingual surface like a greasy or curdy coating.

Hot or irritating edibles may redden the tongue; smoking may dye the tongue greyish and make it dry; breathing through one's mouth during sleep also make the tongue dry. Moreover, scraping of the tongue may change a thick coating into a thin one. Generally, before breakfast, the coating is thicker; after breakfast, it becomes thinner.

If the state of lingual coating is not in accordance with the disease condition, the above-mentioned circumstances should be considered, ascertained, and differentiated.

In order to find out the real states of lingual coating, such as its humidity and firmness, a scraping test may be carried out by using a spatula. This should be performed by scraping the tongue slowly from its root to its tip with moderate strength for 3～5 times. Loose, superficial coatings are easily scraped off; greasy and thick ones are not.

4. Inspection of the tongue proper

1) Vitality

Vitality of a tongue is reflected mainly in its appearance and motility. A flourishing and agile tongue forebodes a good outcome; a withered and stiff tongue forebodes an ominous outcome.

2) Colour

① Pale red tongue generally indicates the deficiency of Vital Energy and Blood. It is often seen in patients suffering from anemia, parasitic infestation, etc.

② Red tongue generally signifies a heat syndrome. Redness merely occurs at the tip of the tongue signifies the flaming up of Heart Fire; redness at lateral sides of the tongue signifies Liver-Gallbladder Fire; redness at the middle of the tongue signifies the damage of Stomach Yin.

Red tongue with blood spots signifies the damage of Pericardium by Heat; red tongue with petechia signifies the exhibition of petechia all over the body.

Bright red tongue signifies extreme Heat in epidemic febrile disease; it may also signify the deficiency of Yin in consumptive disease.

③ Crimson or deep red tongue generally signifies the exuberance of Heat, or Nutrient System has been invaded.

Crimson tongue with sticky and greasy coating signifies Turbidity is involved in the disease.

Crimson tongue with yellowish white coating signifies the Warm evil has not left Energy System completely.

Crimson tongue with a dry surface in the middle part signifies an exuberance of Stomach Fire and the exhaustion of body fluids.

Bright crimson tongue signifies Pericardium is invaded.

Glossy crimson tongue signifies the depletion of Stomach Yin.

Dim crimson tongue which is dried and withered signifies the depletion of Kidney Yin.

④ Purple and tumid tongue signifies the offending of Heart by alcoholic toxin.

Dim purple tongue generally signifies the accumulation of stagnated Blood.

Moist, slippery, purple tongue signifies a Yin syndrome resulting from a direct attack on Liver-Kidney.

Purple tongue with dry and yellow coating signifies long-cherished Heat, especially in Spleen-Stomach.

⑤ A coated blue tongue signifies the disease condition may be remedied, although Viscera have been damaged.

Slight blue which has not spread over the whole tongue may be seen in patients suffering from pestilence or Heat stagnation in Wetness-Warm.

Blue tongue with slippery, greasy coating signifies Yin evil has converted into Heat.

Glossy blue tongue without coating signifies the extreme depletion of Vital Energy and Blood, a critical condition.

3) Appearance

Solid, dark coloured tongue generally signifies a sthenic syndrome; tender, light coloured tongue generally signifies an asthenic syndrome.

Stiff tongue is usually seen in patients suffering from apoplexy, or high fever with impairment of consciousness, or with loss of Fluid.

Plump tongue or a tongue with teeth prints may be caused by water infiltration, excessive Phlegm due to Spleen asthenia, or upward accumulation of Wetness-Heat.

Thin, emaciated, shrivelled tongue may be caused by Heart Asthenia, Blood deficiency, or waste of soft tissue due to internal Heat.

Swollen, stiff tongue which is red or purple in colour and without pain is usually caused by the hyperactivity of Heart Fire, or the accumulation of Heat in Heart and Spleen.

Shortened, contracted tongue which is unable to protrude, is usually caused by Cold, Heat, Wetness, or Phlegm.

Curled tongue with ascended testes is a critical sign of the complete exhaustion of Liver Meridian Energy, usually seen in the terminal stage of an acute febrile disease or in severe cerebrovascular accidents.

Glossy tongue without coating, or mirror-like tongue, signifies an extreme exhaustion of Stomach Yin.

Fissured tongue is a sign of Yin Asthenia caused by protracted illness.

Double tongue may be a congenital deformity, tumour, sublingual fibroma, or inflammation of the sublingual soft tissue.

Sores of the tongue are exceedingly painful; they vary in size, number, and distribution. Sores jutting from the lingual surface usually signifies an upward attack of Heart Fire. Sores sunken below the lingual surface usually signifies the flaring up of asthenic Fire due to the deficiency of Liver-Kidney Yin.

4) Motility

Wry tongue indicates a tongue turning to one side when it is protruded. It is usually seen in apoplexy.

Tremor of the tongue is usually caused by internal Wind or alcoholism.

Sluggish tongue or retracted tongue implies it is curled and stiff, thereby sluggish in moving and difficult in speaking. This is usually due to the obstruction of Heart Aperture by Phlegm, or the depletion of Yin by Heat, commonly seen in apoplexy, epidemic meningitis, encephalitis B, and their sequelae.

Playing with the tongue implies a morbid condition marked by extending the tongue out and drawing it back frequently, or licking the lips and corners of the mouth. It signifies the exuberance of Heat in Heart and Spleen generally. It is also an omen of convulsion and poor mental development in infants.

Wagging tongue implies the tongue is relaxed, lengthened, and protruded out of the mouth. It is usually seen in children suffering from cerebral hypoplasia, or febrile disease when CNS is involved.

Flaccid tongue which is weak and unable to curl and protrude, signifies the extreme exhaustion of Vital Energy and Blood, or the depletion of Yin and Fluid.

Numb tongue with ineffective motility is generally due to the deficiency of both Vital Energy and Blood.

5. Inspection of the lingual coating

Under normal circumstances, there is a layer of white, thin, and furlike substance covering the lingual surface which is moist, clean, and lively.

1) Colour

① White: White coating generally signifies an exterior or cold syndrome. White, thin, and slippery coating signifies an exopathy caused by Wind-Cold. White, slippery, and sticky coating generally signifies the existence of internal Wetness-Phlegm. White, tender, and slippery coating which can be scraped completely signifies an interior asthenic cold syndrome. White coating on a crimson tongue signifies the containment of Wetness by hidden Heat. White coating like a layer of accumulated white powder signifies serious filthy Turbidity in epidemic febrile diseases. White, thick, dry, and cracked coating with sharply contoured granules like sand may be caused by sudden and violent onset of internal Heat accompanied with extreme exhaustion of body fluids. Under such circumstances, there is no time for the coating to change from white colour to yellow colour.

② Yellow: Yellow coating generally signifies an interior heat syndrome. The deeper the yellow, the higher the heat. Light yellow coating which is still moist, signifies the exopathic evil begins to invade the interior. Yellow, thick, dry coating signifies the exuberance of internal heat and body fluids has been consumed. Scorchingly yellow, dry, and cracked coating signifies the extreme exuberance of internal heat and body fluids have been depleted. Under such circumstances, the tongue may be prickled. Yellow, slippery, and greasy coating signifies the accumulation of Wetness-Heat in Spleen-Stomach, or internal heat complicated by Phlegm-Turbidity. Light yellow, moist coating signifies the decline of Yang and the debility of Spleen.

③ Grey: Grey colour, in other words, is light black. Generally, grey coating signifies an interior syndrome. Grey and dry coating signifies the exuberance of Heat and the depletion of body fluids. Grey and moist coating signifies an internal obstruction due to Cold-Wetness.

④ Black: Black coating may signify an extreme internal Heat or an extreme internal Cold, and it often appears in critical stage. Black, dry, cracked, or prickled coating generally signifies an extreme Heat and Genuine Yin is about to be dried up. Black, moist, slippery coating generally signifies the existence of obstinate Cold-Wetness. Other colours may also be seen occasionally. Lingual coating of different colours may be seen at different parts of the same tongue. Dynamic changes from one colour to another signify the dynamic changes of nature and location of syndromes correspondingly.

2) Thickness:

From the thickness of lingual coating, we may assess the invading depth of pathogenic evils and the developing trend of a clinical course. Thin coating generally signifies a mild disorder, Healthy Energy has not been damaged, an exterior syndrome, or the condition is not serious.

Thick coating generally signifies a serious disorder, the exuberance of pathogenic evils, an interior syndrome, or the accumulation of Phlegm, Wetness, Turbidity, or the retention of body fluids or food.

When a lingual coating changes from thin to thick, it generally signifies an advance of disease. When a lingual coating changes from thick to thin, it generally signifies a retreat of disease.

3) Humidity

Moistness and dryness of lingual coating reflect the wax and wane of body fluids.

Moist coating generally signifies body fluids have not been damaged. Slippery coating generally signifies Wetness, Cold, or the upward outflow of Phlegm-Fluid resulting from the decline of Yang or Vital Energy.

Dry coating generally signifies the exuberance of Heat, the exhaustion of Yin or Fluid, or the failure of upward transportation of Fluid due to Yang or Vital Energy debility. When a coating changes from moist to dry, or vice versa, it generally signifies a change of pathologic state correspondingly.

4) Quality

Corroded coating is thick, loose, like bean dregs, easy to be wiped away. It generally signifies the retention of food, or the accumulation of Phlegm or Turbidity.

Greasy coating is slimy, like an oily layer, unable to be wiped away or scraped off. It generally signifies Wetness-Turbidity, Phlegm, or food retention.

5) Distribution

A complete coating covers the entire lingual surface. It generally signifies a diffuse invasion of pathogenic evils.

A partial coating may be at the anterior, posterior, medial, or lateral of the lingual surface. Clinical significance of various types of distribution has already been mentioned in *Distribution of Internal Organs on Lingual Surface*.

6) Peeling off of the lingual coating

This is invariably caused by the depletion of both Stomach Energy and Stomach Yin.

If a piece of thick coating peels off, exposing a reddened, dry lingual surface, it is an ominous omen.

If the peeling off occurs at multiple sites with clear-cut margins exposing the lingual surface, it is called a *Geographic Tongue*.

If a coating peels off entirely, it is called a mirror-like tongue.

7) Rooted or superficial

Coatings which are rooted, tight, unable to be scraped away, are genuine ones; those which are superficial, loose, easy to be scraped away, are pseudo ones.

A genuine coating signifies the dominance of pathogenic evil, the existence of Stomach Energy, or a favourable prognosis.

A pseudo coating signifies an asthenic or cold syndrome in protracted illness, the impending exhaustion of Stomach Energy, or an ominous prognosis.

8) Growing or declining

A coating changes from thick to thin generally signifies a gradual convalescence or the retreat of illness. A coating changes from thin to thick generally signifies a gradual dominance of pathogenic evil or the advance of illness.

Sudden growth of coating signifies a swift decline of Health Energy; sudden decline of coating signifies a swift exhaustion of Stomach Energy.

Regardless of growth or decline, a gradual change of coating implies a favourable prognosis; a sudden change implies an ominous prognosis.

ANNEX Inspection of Sublingual Vessel Collaterals

This is a new method of diagnostic examination developed in recent years. Sublingual Vessel Collaterals stem from the base of the tongue and connect directly with Viscera, especially Heart, Spleen, Liver, and Kidney. Under normal circumstances, they are bluish purple in colour and moist; they travel naturally, without meandering, distending, or varicosity.

1. Appearance

1) Distending or engorged Collaterals signify Blood stasis which may be caused either by internal Heat or by internal Cold.

If such Collaterals are bright bluish purple and dry, they signify the exuberance of Heat and depletion of body fluids.

If such Collaterals are dim bluish purple with abundant saliva, they signify the dominance of Cold.

2) Tortuosity or varicosity

Tortuous Collaterals with normal colour and lustre signify the stagnation of Liver Energy commonly seen in females.

Varicose and cyanotic Collaterals generally signify Vital Energy stagnation and Blood stasis, or blockage of Collaterals.

Tortuous, shrivelled with less moistened Collaterals signify the damage of Yin caused by long-standing internal Heat or Vital Energy depression.

3) Thin or slender Collaterals generally signify Blood or Yin deficiency.

Thin, purple Collaterals with scanty saliva generally signify the consumption of body fluids by asthenic Fire, or the hyperactivity of Fire due to Yin deficiency.

2. Colour

1) Cyanotic colour of sublingual Collaterals generally signifies Heat, Cold, or Blood stasis.

Cyanotic, thick Collaterals signify the exuberance of Heat.

Cyanotic, thin Collaterals signify the damage of Fluid by excessive Heat.

Moist, distending, cyanotic Collaterals signify the exuberance of Cold, the debility of Yang, or the retention of Phlegm-Wetness or Fluid.

Tortuous Collaterals with unevenly spread cyanotic colour signify Vital Energy stagnation and Blood stasis.

2) Black colour of sublingual Collaterals generally signifies an extreme Heat or an extreme Cold.

Shrivelled tongue with dry, thin sublingual Collaterals generally signifies an extreme Heat. Under these circumstances, most patients can not stick up their tongues and it is necessary to use a spatula.

Plump tongue with moist, thick sublingual Collaterals generally signifies an Extreme Cold. Under these circumstances, some patients can still stick up their tongues to facilitate the examination.

There are some limitations of this new method of diagnostic examination. For instance, children are often non-cooperative; patients with stiff tongue, flaccid tongue, or wry tongue, etc; cannot stick up their tongues; and the examination may be impossible even by using a spatula.

6. Relationship between inspection of the tongue proper, its coating, and its sublingual Collaterals.

Generally speaking, their manifestations are consistent with each other. For instance, crimson tongue with yellow coating and cyanotic sublingual Collaterals indicates a sthenic heat syndrome. But pathologic changes are intricate and variable. Sometimes manifestations of the tongue proper, its coating, and its sublingual Collaterals may be inconsistent. For example, in a syndrome of Blood stasis, changes of sublingual Collaterals are more sensitive than those of the tongue proper, while its coating remains as usual. In a syndrome of Wetness-Heat, there may be a crimson tongue with white and greasy coating. When Wetness-Heat is accumulated and condensed in Spleen-Stomach, there may be yellow and coarse coating at the periphery of the tongue, greyish black, thick, and greasy coating in the middle part, yet the change of the tongue proper is not significant.

In short, various manifestations in different aspects of the tongue should be examined meticulously and assessed comprehensively by taking all factors into consideration.

V. *Inspection of the head, neck, Five Sense Organs, and Lower Apertures*

According to theories of Meridians, Tendons, and Outward Manifestations of Viscera, "All Yang Meridians meet at the head"; and Five Sense Organs and Lower Apertures are connected with internal organs through Meridians and Collaterals, as well as Tendon Meridians.

1. Inspection of the head and face
1) Shape
Inspection of the shape of the patient's head contributes to the evaluation of his (her) level of intelligence, as well as his (her) vicissitude of Kidney Essence.

① Macrocephalia: This is characterized by bulging fontanel and prominent forehead, triangular face, setting-sun eyes; the size of the head is out of proportion with the body. There is infantile metopismus or congenital hydrocephalus concurrently.

② Microcephalia: This is characterized by sunken fontanel, infantile metopismus, and mental retardation, and is generally caused by congenital defects or the deficiency of Kidney Essence.

③ Cephalus quadratus: This may be accompanied with Five Kinds of Retardation: Retarded standing, walking, hair-growing, tooth eruption, and speaking faculty.

④ Bulging of the fontanel: In epidemic febrile disease of infants, this may be caused by the upward attack of evil Fire, or the pathologic change in the brain. But the bulging of fontanel is a normal phenomenon when infants cry.

2) Head shaking

Involuntary head shaking generally signifies a disorder caused by Wind, or by the exhaustion of both Vital Energy and Blood.

3) Facial edema

This is commonly seen in hydropsy. Yang hydropsy develops quite swiftly and begins at the eyelids and the face. Yin hydropsy develops rather slowly and begins at the feet and legs. Sudden onset of burning hotness and swelling of the head with a flushed face indicates an upward attack of virulent Fire from Wind-Heat. If the head and face are seriously swollen, as a result the patient cannot open his (her) eyes, it may be an "infection with swollen head" caused by virulent Fire from seasonal pestilence.

4) Swelling of the cheek

This indicates the sudden swelling of the cheek on one side or both sides, often accompanied with flushed face, sore throat, even deafness.

5) Deviation of the eye and mouth

The eye and the corner of the mouth on the diseased side cannot be closed. The patient cannot frown his (her) eyebrows or bloat his (her) cheeks. This generally signifies an attack of Wind evil on the basis of Collateral voidness or Collaterals are blocked by Wind-Phlegm.

2. Inspection of the hair

Black, thick, sleek, and glossy hair signifies the abundance of Blood and Kidney Essence.

Dry, sparse, or withered hair and hair falling generally signify the deficiency of Kidney Essence.

Alopecia areata (single or multiple) signifies an attack of Wind on the basis of Blood Asthenia.

Thin, sparse hair and the liability of its falling in young or middle-aged people are generally due to Blood Heat or Kidney Asthenia.

Hair entangled like tassels is a sign of infantile malnutrition.

3. Inspection of the neck and nape

1) Goiter

According to TCM, this is generally caused by the depression of Vital Energy and the accumulation and condensation of Phlegm.

2) Scrofula

According to TCM, this is called Phlegm nodule or Phlegm nodules. It is caused by the scorching effect of asthenic Fire induced by Yin deficiency.

3) Stiff neck or opisthotonus

This generally signifies the upward assault of Evil Fire in epidemic febrile disease, or the upward attack of Wind-Fire in apoplexy.

4) Flaccid nape with drooping head

This is a sign of the exhaustion of Vital Essence.

4. Inspection of the eye

According to the theory of Five Orbiculi, different parts of the eye belong to corresponding Parenchymatous Viscera. These are shown in the following table.

Orbiculus	Anatomic site	Parenchymatous Viscera
Blood	canthus	Heart
Wind	the black of the eye	Liver
Energy	the white of the eye	Lung
Water	pupil	Kidney
Flesh	eyelid	Spleen

Table 1. Relationship between Five Orbiculi and Five Parenchymatous Viscera

1) Vitality

See also "Inspection of expression, vitality, and mental state" in Section 1, Chapter II.

2) Colour

① Conjunctival congestion with swelling and pain generally signifies a sthenic heat syndrome. Redness occurring at the white of the eye signifies Lung Heat. Redness occurring at the canthus signifies Heart Fire. Redness occurring all over the eye signifies Wind-Heat in Liver Meridian. Marginal blepharitis is caused by Wetness-Heat and/or Spleen Fire.

② Pale conjunctiva and canthus signify Blood deficiency.

③ Yellow conjunctiva and sclera signify the fuming and steaming of Wetness-Heat, or jaundice in current medicine.

3) Shape

① Puffiness of eyelids is a sign of early hydropsy. Edema of lower eyelids in the aged signifies the deficiency of Kidney Energy and the decline of Kidney Yang. Sometimes transient, slight eyelid edema may occur in healthy people after a sound sleep.

② Sunken orbit is generally due to the depletion of body fluids or the deficiency of Vital Energy and Blood. If eyeballs sink in their orbits and the patient loses his (her) sight, it is an omen of the exhaustion of both Yin and Yang.

③ Exophthalmus with dyspnea suggests the fullness and distension of Lung. Exophthalmus with swelling of the neck suggests goiter. Sudden protruding of a single eyeball signifies an ominous outcome.

④ Nebula generally belongs to an external ophthalmopathy.

⑤ Deformed pupils or visual disturbance with a normal appearance of eyes belongs to an internal ophthalmopathy.

⑥ Pterygium is generally caused by the exuberance of Wind-Heat in Heart and Lung Meridians, or the steaming and clogging action of Wetness-Heat in Spleen-Stomach. This may also be caused by the flaming up of Heart Fire as a result of Liver-Kidney Yin deficiency.

⑦ Miosis is generally due to the blazing of Liver-Gallbladder Fire in apoplexy, the upward attack of virulent Warm-Heat in epidemic febrile disease, or the intoxication of Radix Aconiti, Radix Aconiti Kusnezoffii, etc.

⑧ Mydriasis is generally caused by the depletion of Kidney Essence, a critical sign just before dying. It may also occur in glaucoma caused by the upward harassment of Wind-Fire in Liver-Gallbladder, or in Datura intoxication.

4) Eyeball position and motility.

① Superduction or strabismus is generally caused by the upstirring of Liver Wind.

② Lethargy with eyes half-closed is generally due to the debility of Spleen Energy, or the failure in uprising of Lucid Yang.

③ Slightly fixed eyeballs are generally caused by the internal obstruction of Phlegm-Heat.

In short, superduction, staring blankly forward, mydriasis, hyperphoria with fixed eyeballs and opisthotonus are critical signs.

5. Inspection of the ear

According to TCM, *Kidney has its specific orifice in the ear;* and various Meridians connect with the ear, such as Three Yang Meridians of the Hand and Foot, Jueyin Meridian of the Hand, etc. Therefore, the ear is closely linked with various Viscera and all parts of the body. Spots with tenderness or with changes of electric resistance may be detected on the auricle, reflecting disorders of different locales correspondingly. There may be even changes of colour, appearance, such as blister, nodule, papula, and desquamation at corresponding spots.

As to details of inspection of the ear, please refer to an atlas of Auricular Points.

6. Inspection of the nose

The nose is the opening of Lung. It belongs to Spleen Meridian and is associated with Stomach Meridian, etc.

1) Colour

Pale nasal apex signifies a loss of blood; yellow colour of the nose signifies an exuberance of Wetness-Heat; blue colour signifies abdominal pain; red colour signifies Heat in Spleen and Lung; light black signifies the retention of body fluids; black and dried nostrils signify an extreme Heat.

2) Appearance

Rosacea signifies Blood Heat in Lung. Ulceration and collapse of the nasal column generally signify an upward attack of malicious evil. Flaring of nares signifies the existence of difficulty in breathing or the impending exhaustion of Lung Energy.

3) Secretion

Clear snivel signifies an attack of Wind-Cold; turbid snivel signifies an attack of Wind-Heat; stench, purulent snivel signifies sinusitis.

7. Inspection of the mouth and lips

The mouth is the opening of Spleen which flourishes at lips. Moreover, Yangming Meridian of the Hand and Foot revolves around the mouth.

1) Colour

Ruddy lips signify that Stomach Energy is exuberant. Pale lips signify the deficiency of both Vital Energy and Blood; deep red lips signify a heat syndrome; deep red and dry lips signify an exuberance of Heat and the depletion of Yin. Cyanotic lips suggest the stagnation of Blood circulation. Black colour around the mouth suggests the exhaustion of Kidney Energy. Black, dry, and curled lips are an ominous sign of Spleen failure.

2) Appearance

Dry mouth with cracked lips signifies Fluid deficiency; erosion of the mouth and lips signifies Wetness-Heat in Spleen-Stomach; redness, hotness, swelling, itching, or pain of the mouth and lips signify an upward assault of Stomach Fire.

Twitching of the oral corner suggests the stirring of Liver Wind; deviation of the mouth and eyes suggests facial paralysis or apoplexy; Neonatal lockjaw indicates tetanus of the newborn.

Aphtha is generally caused by accumulated Heat in Heart-Spleen; mycotic stomatitis or thrush is due to hidden Heat in Heart-Spleen.

Slobbering along corner of the mouth generally indicates the debility of Spleen.

8. Inspection of the gum and teeth

Kidney is in charge of the bone, The teeth are the odds and ends of the bone. According to TCM, Yangming Meridian of the Hand and Foot terminates in the gum.

Pale gum indicates Blood deficiency; withered gum may be caused by an exuberance of Heat, the depletion of Yin, or the exhaustion of Essence and Vital Energy; swelling, pain, and bleeding of the gum signify an injury of Collaterals by Stomach Heat; bleeding of the gum without swelling and pain suggests an injury of Collaterals by asthenic Fire.

Pale and shrivelled gum with wizened teeth signifies the exhaustion of Kidney Yin; slackened teeth with exposed dental roots signify the flaming up of asthenic Fire due to the deficiency of Kidney Yin; delayed growth of permanent teeth in children indicates the deficiency of Kidney Energy; teeth grinding in sleep suggests dyspepsia, Stomach Heat, or parasitic infestation; involuntary teeth gnashing may be a sign of Liver Wind; trismus is commonly due to the obstruction of Collaterals by Wind-Phlegm, or stirring of Wind by exuberant Heat.

Ulcerative gingivitis with teeth dropping is an ominous sign.

9. Inspection of the throat

The pharynx communicates with Stomach, the larynx communicates with Lung. Thus the throat is a passageway of ingested diet and respiratory gas. Various Meridians connect with the throat; among them, Kidney Meridian travels along it and embraces the lingual base from both sides.

1) Swelling, pain, and ulceration

Redness, swelling, and pain of the throat, sometimes accompanied with ulceration and yellowish white pus, signify an upward assault of Virulent Heat. Tender redness with slight pain, or dry redness without swelling signifies the flaming up of asthenic Fire on the basis of Yin deficiency. Pale redness with diffuse swelling signifies the accumulation and stagnation of Phlegm-Wetness.

2) Pseudomembrane

Sometimes there is a pseudomembrane which covers the ulcerated lesion. Generally, it is thick, loosened, and apt to be wiped away. After being wiped away, it does not recur. Such pseudomembrane is usually caused by the exuberance and clogging of Stomach Heat.

Greyish white, firm, tenacious, and evenly distributed pseudomembrane which is difficult to be peeled off, signifies diphtheria. According to TCM. it is due to the damage of Yin by Dryness-Fire generally. When such pseudomembrane is peeled off, bleeding occurs.

10. Inspection of the lower apertures

This includes the inspection of the urino-genital aperture (external genitalia) and the anus.

Kidney has its specific opening in the urino-genital aperture and the anus. The external genitalia is closely related to most Viscera and Meridians, especially Liver. Besides Kidney, the anus is related to Lung, Spleen, Stomach, and Large Intestine.

1) The external genitalia

Swollen scrotum without itching and pain is generally caused by the downward overflow of Water-Wetness. Swelling and distension of labia without pain generally indicate hydropsy. Enlarged, soft scrotum may be a sign of inguinal hernia. Redness, hotness, swelling, and pain of the testis or testes are generally due to Wetness-Heat in Liver Meridian. Hard, tumescent testis without redness and hotness signifies a cold syndrome or a deficiency of Vital Energy. Drawing back of the testis or testes into the abdomen is generally caused by the condensing effect of Cold. Prolapse of the uterus is generally due to the deficiency and collapse of Spleen Energy.

2) The anus

Painful anal fissure, which bleeds during defecation, is generally due to the accumulation of Heat in Large Intestine, or the extrusion of stercoroma. Hemorrhoid and anal fistula are generally due to a mixed invasion of Wetness-Heat-Wind-Dryness. Prolapse of the rectum is generally due to the debility and collapse of Vital Energy.

VI. *Inspection of the skin*

The skin is associated with Lung, and contributes to the body resistance guarding against exopathic evils. Significance and implications of skin inspection are the same as those of the facial complexion. Moreover, the following skin eruptions should be watched for:

1. Pea-shaped eruption

1) Smallpox

The eruption of smallpox is characterized by circular shape, crimson base, and a depressed apex like a navel. Eruptions of smallpox occur simultaneously and are of the same size, followed by pustulation, sloughing, and scar formation.

2) Varicella

The eruption of varicella is a vesicle with clear content, but without areola at its base and a depression at its apex. Eruptions of varicella occur irregularly and are of various size. There are no sloughing and no scar formation.

2. Macula and exanthem

Maculae are patchy and flat; exanthems are millet-shaped and protruding.

1) Maculae

① Yang maculae: Yang maculae are ruddy and scattered, commonly seen in acute febrile diseases caused by epidemic Warm-Heat. They signify that Nutrient and Blood Systems have been invaded. When maculae become crimson or purplish black and dense, accompanied with ardent fever and unconsciousness, it signifies an inward encroachment of pathogenic evils.

② Yin maculae: Yin maculae are pale red or dim purple, capricious, and distributed sparsely. They are generally caused by the damage of Interior or the deficiency of Vital Energy and Blood. Patients are sober-minded, accompanied with various asthenic syndromes.

2) Exanthem

① Measles: Measles is an acute infectious disease in children caused by seasonal epidemic evils invading Lung and Stomach. It is characterized by cough, conjunctival congestion, photophobia, and eyes brimming with tears at the beginning. Measles emerge firstly at the back of ears, the hairline, the neck, and then spread gradually over the trunk and other parts of the body. They are pink in colour with distinct demarkation.

② Rubella: Rubella is caused by seasonal Wind-Heat invading Lung and Defence System. During eruption, there are cough and an itching sensation generally. Eruptions disappear within 2~3 days.

③ Urticaria: Urticaria is characterized by raised edematous patches with distinct demarkation and accompanied with intolerable intense itching. It may be caused by Wind-Heat, Wind-Cold, or Wind-Wetness. Protracted urticaria is generally due to the deficiency of Vital Energy and Blood.

3. Miliaria alba, herpes zoster, and eczema

1) Miliaria alba

Miliaria alba or sudamina crystallina is caused by Wetness-Warm. Its eruptions are white, small vesicles with clear watery content, emerging over the neck, chest, or abdomen. When they are glittering, translucent, and plump, these signify a favourable outcome. When they are withered, it signifies the exhaustion of Vital Energy and body fluids, or the inward encroachment of pathogenic evils.

2) Herpes zoster

Burning hot sensation and stabbing pain at the local part on body surface, such as the chest, hypochondria, back, etc. Vesicles of various sizes are clustered with red halos. This is generally due to the fumigating and steaming action of Wetness-Heat caused by Liver-Gallbladder Fire.

3) Eczema

At first, it looks like an erythema. Thereafter it swells and distends, or blisters. Blisters rupture before long, oozing mucus, resulting in red erosions. After several or tens of days, it becomes dried and crusted. After decrustation, a red vestige remains and disppears gradually. This is generally caused by Wind-Wetness-Heat on the basis of weakness of Healthy Energy.

4. Inspection of carbuncle, cellulitis, and furuncle
1) Carbuncle

This indicates a painfull local purulentinflammation of the skin and deeper tissues with multiple openings for the discharge of pus. It is generally caused by the accumulation of virulent Fire and Wetness-Heat, accompanied with Vital Energy stagnation and Blood stasis, resulting in tissue sloughing.

2) Cellulitis

This is characterized by diffuse swelling and slight pain at the local part, where there are no purulent core, no change of skin colour, and no sensation of hotness. It is a Yin syndrome and is generally caused by the stagnation and condensation of Cold-Phlegm on the basis of Vital Energy and Blood deficiency.

3) Furuncle

Furuncle is small, round, and superficial. Its swelling and pain are not serious. It is softened after suppuration and healed after its diabrosis. Furuncle generally occurs multiply, rising one after another. It is often caused by the accumulation of Summer-Heat and Wetness.

4) Malignant boil

Malignant boil begins with a small apex like a millet, and a hardened deep root. There are numbness, itching, and pain at the local part. It is generally caused by the sudden attack of virulent evils, resulting in stagnation and condensation of Vital Energy and Blood.

If a red streak appears from the boil and extends centripetally and swiftly, it is called a *red-streaked infection*, or *carbuncle complicated by septicemia* which signifies the impending attack of virulent evils on internal organs.

VII. *Inspection of Superficial Venules of the Index Finger (SVIF)*

Superficial Venules of the Index Finger branch off from Taiyin Meridian. Their inspection corresponds to the pulse taking in adults and it is suitable for children under 3 years of age. SVIF is divided into three parts in line with the three segments of the index finger and they are named Three Passes.

1. Three Passes

These indicate Wind Pass, Energy Pass, and Vital Pass.

Wind Pass: The proximal segment of the index finger.

Energy Pass: The intermediate segment of the index finger.

Vital Pass: The distal segment of the index finger.

2. Technique of inspection

Under sufficient illumination in broad day, hold the child's index finger with the thumb and index finger of the left hand, inspect its SVIF; or push the child's index finger from Vital Pass, through Energy Pass, to Wind Pass with the thumb of the right hand for several times, to make SVIF evident.

3. Pathologic manifestations of SVIF

When SVIF appears at Wind Pass, it signifies a mild or superficial disease. When SVIF penetrates through Wind Pass and enters into Energy Pass, it signifies a serious disease. If SVIF enters into Vital Pass, even reaches to the finger-nail, it signifies a critical condition.

If SVIF lengthens day by day, it signifies a deteriorating disease condition. If SVIF shortens day by day, it signifies an improving disease condition.

Thickening of SVIF signifies a heat or sthenic syndrome; thinning of SVIF signifies a cold or asthenic syndrome.

Superficial and evident SVIF signifies an exterior syndrome; deep and hidden SVIF signifies an interior syndrome.

Bright red SVIF signifies an exterior syndrome caused by Wind-Cold generally; purplish red SVIF signifies an interior heat syndrome; pale yellow SVIF signifies the debility of Spleen; blue SVIF signifies Wind or pain; purplish black SVIF signifies the blockage of Blood circulation.

Pale and lustreless SVIF signifies an asthenic syndrome, such as the deficiency of Vital Energy and Blood; deep, dim coloured and stagnated SVIF signifies a sthenic syndrome, such as the accumulation of Phlegm-Fire.

VIII. *Inspection of various discharge*

Discharge includes excreta and secreta. Generally speaking, white, clear, unformed discharge signifies the damage of Yang or a cold syndrome; yellow, thick, formed discharge signifies the simmering of Fluid by Heat or a heat syndrome.

1. Inspection of phlegm and nasal discharge

1) Clear, dilute, frothy phlegm accompanied with dizziness, oppressed feeling in the chest, etc., generally signifies Wind-Phlegm.

2) White, slippery, abundant phlegm which is apt to be expectorated, generally signifies Wetness-Phlegm.

3) Scanty, sticky phlegm which is difficult to be expectorated, signifies Dryness-Phlegm.

4) Phlegm tinged with bright red blood generally signifies the damage of Lung Collaterals by Heat.

5) Stench phlegm with pus and blood generally signifies pulmonary abscess.

6) Turbid nasal discharge signifies an exogenic attack of Wind-Heat; clear nasal discharge signifies an exogenic attack of Wind-Cold. Protracted, incessant, turbid nasal discharge signifies nasal sinusitis.

2. Inspection of saliva and spittle

1) Incessant, clear slobbering generally signifies Spleen Asthenia or a cold syndrome of Spleen. Sticky spittle which may be drawn like candies floss, generally signifies Wetness-Heat in Spleen-Stomach.

2) Involuntary slobbering, especially during sleep, is generally due to the debility of Spleen, parasitic infestation, or Stomach Heat in children.

3) Spitting of copious frothy saliva generally signifies Wetness-Cold in Stomach, or the debility of Kidney Yang.

3. Inspection of vomitus

1) Clear, dilute vomitus without acid and offensive odour generally signifies an asthenic and cold syndrome of Stomach.

2) Filthy, turbid, sour, stinking vomitus generally signifies a sthenic and heat syndrome of Stomach.

3) Sour and putrid vomitus with undigested food generally signifies dyspepsia caused by over-eating or improper diet.

4) Yellowish green, bitter, watery vomitus generally signifies depressed Heat in Liver-Gallbladder.

5) Spitting of bright red or dim purple blood mixed with food residue generally signifies the damage of Stomach Collaterals.

Section 2. Auscultation and Smelling

I. *Auscultation*

1. Voice

Variation of voice may reflect the nature of illness and the vicissitude of Healthy Energy.

1) Loudness of voice

A sonorous voice accompanied with talkativeness generally signifies a sthenic and/or heat syndrome; a low and timid voice accompanied with laziness of speaking generally signifies an asthenic and / or a cold syndrome.

2) Change of intonation

Heavy and coarse voice or speaking with a twang is generally due to a restraint of Exterior by Wind-Cold, or the obstruction of Lung Energy.

3) Groaning

Incessant groaning generally signifies pain. Groaning while one presses his (her) chest or abdomen generally signifies chest or abdominal pain.

4) Husky voice or aphonia

When they occur in a newly diseased patient, generally they signify a sthenic syndrome, such as caused by an attack of exogenous Wind-Cold or Wind-Heat. When they occur in a protracted disease, generally they signify an asthenic syndrome, such as caused by the deficiency of Lung-

Kidney Yin, or the scorching effect of asthenic Fire on Lung.

Moreover, exhaustive shouting may result in husky voice or aphonia due to the depletion of Vital Energy and Yin. Aphonia during pregnancy may be caused by the blockage of Collaterals due to fetal oppression, which connect with the throat and the lingual base.

2. Speech

1) Taciturnity

Taciturnity generally signifies an asthenic, cold syndrome; fretfulness and talkativeness generally signify a sthenic, heat syndrome.

2) Fading murmuring

This indicates absent-mindedness, repetition of speech, speaking from time to time with low and feeble voice. Generally, this signifies an asthenic syndrome, such as caused by the exhaustion of Essence from protracted illness, the malnourishment of Heart, etc.

3) Delirium

This indicates unconsciousness and inconsequential talk with a loud and energetic voice. Generally, this signifies a sthenic syndrome, such as caused by the encroachment on Pericardium by Warm-Heat in epidemic febrile diseases; or a sthenic syndrome of Hollow Viscera, such as Yangming Stomach, in Exogenous Febrile Disease.

4) Soliloquy

This indicates talking to oneself ceaselessly and incoherently. If the patient knows what he (she) had said, it is a sign of paraphasia. Both soliloquy and paraphasia signify an Yin syndrome, or an obstruction of Heart Aperture by Phlegm condensation, etc.

5) Ravings

Laughing, cursing, talking wildly, or singing loudly on an upland, throwing away clothes, and rushing about signify a Yang syndrome, such as caused by Phlegm-Fire harassing the normal function of Heart, etc.

6) Soft, slow, and feeble talk and longing to speak but failure to repeat the speech signify an asthenic syndrome, or an extreme exhaustion of Spleen-Stomach Energy.

7) Dysphasia

Dysphasia signifies the covering up of Lucid Aperture by Wind-Phlegm, or the obstruction of Vessel Collaterals by Wind-Phlegm.

3. Respiratory sound

Lung is in charge of Vital Energy; Kidney governs the reception of air. Therefore according to TCM, abnormalities of respiration reflect the pathologic changes of lung and kidney primarily.

1) Breath

① Feeble breath: Feeble breath signifies an asthenic or a cold syndrome, and is generally caused by an internal damage or the deficiency of Vital Energy.

② Gruff breath: Gruff breath signifies a sthenic or a heat syndrome, and is generally caused by an exopathic attack.

③ Shortness of breath: This indicates short, rapid, and interrupted breathing without anguish or lifting of shoulders. It is generally due to the debility of Lung Energy or the retention of Fluid in the chest.

④ Deficiency of breath: This indicates a faint and short breath with a low respiratory sound and normal body posture, and is generally due to the deficiency of Primordial Energy, or the debility of Middle Energizer.

2) Gasping

Gasping indicates dyspnea with urgency and shortness of breath, even mouth breathing with lifting shoulders and flaring nares. The patient is generally unable to lie flat in bed. This may be classified as the sthenic and the asthenic.

① Sthenic gasping: This indicates sudden and violent onset of loud respiratory sound and gruff breathing, facing upward with protruded eyes. The patient feels relieved only through a satisfactory expiration. Generally, it is due to sthenic Lung Heat, or the retention of Phlegm-Fluid in the chest, etc.

② Asthenic gasping: This is characterized by slow and gradual onset, low respiratory sound, and shortness of breath; symptoms aggravated during physical labour. The patient feels relieved after a full inspiration. This is generally caused by the debility of Lung-kidney

Energy.

3) Bronchial wheezing

This indicates gasping with wheezing caused by the accumulation of phlegm in the air passage, which breaks out now and then. When panting and bronchial wheezing occur simultaneously, it is called "asthma".

4) Heaving sighs

This is generally caused by emotional depression.

5) Abnormal uprising of Vital Energy

This indicates a reversed flow of Vital Energy in the larynx, accompanied with feeling of oppression in the chest, or cough, spitting of glutinous sputum. In serious cases, patients cannot lie flat in bed.

Abnormal uprising of Vital Energy accompanied with hydropsy generally signifies the restraint of Lung by exopathogen, resulting in Water-Fluid retention.

Abnormal uprising of Vital Energy accompanied with sore throat genergally signifies the exuberance of Fire on the basis of Yin deficiency.

4. Cough

Cough is due to the impairment of Lung caused either by an internal damage or by an exopathic evil.

1) Heavy and coarse cough sound with white, clear, and dilute phlegm is generally caused by an attack of exogenous Wind-Cold.

2) Low cough sound with yellow and sticky phlegm is generally caused by an attack of Wind-Dryness-Heat.

3) Loud and sonorous cough sound with paroxysmal onset generally signifies a sthenic syndrome.

4) Paroxysmal and incessant cough with a sound like the cry of an egret at the end of such cough, even accompanied by nausea and vomit, signifies Lung Asthenia or pertussis. This is generally due to the wrestling and cohesion of latent Phlegm and Wind, resulting in an obstruction of air passage.

5) Cough with a clear and crisp sound, little or no phlegm, is generally due to an attack of Dryness-Heat on Lung.

6) Faint coughing sound, aphonia due to protracted cough, or

expectoration of white, frothy sputum generally signifies an asthenic syndrome.

7) Protracted, unproductive cough generally signifies the deficiency of Lung Yin.

8) Aggravation of cough at night generally signifies the deficiency of Kidney Yin; aggravation of cough at day-break generally signifies Spleen debility and the exuberance of Wetness.

5. Vomiting sound

Emesis with sound and vomitus is called vomit; emesis with sound but no vomitus is called retching; emesis without sound but with vomitus is called spitting. All these are due to the impairment of harmonizing and descending function of Stomach, or the adverse uprising of Stomach Energy.

1) Slow emesis with faint sound and clear, dilute vomitus signifies an asthenic or a cold syndrome. This may be caused by the debility of Spleen-Stomach Energy, or the retention of Turbid evil in Stomach.

2) Violent and energetic emesis with a loud sound and the vomitus is mixed with sticky sputum or yellow fluid, generally signify a sthenic, heat syndrome.

Under certain circumstances, the cause of vomit should be ascertained carefully. For instance, in food poisoning, what food had been taken should be investigated; in cholera morbus, vomit and diarrhea break out suddenly and simultaneously; in mental disorder caused by high fever, the vomit is projectile and there is no sensation of nausea before vomit.

6. Hiccup

This indicates an involuntary, loud, high-pitched sound with short duration through the throat caused by an adverse upward rushing of Stomach Energy.

1) Successive, loud, energetic hiccup which breaks out again and again, generally signifies a sthenic, heat syndrome.

2) Low, feeble hiccup which breaks out intermittently and

infrequently generally signifies an asthenic, or a cold syndrome.

3) Sudden onset of hiccup in protracted illness or in a critical condition generally signifies the collapse of Stomach Energy.

7. Eructation

Eructation is also caused by the adverse uprising of Stomach Energy. The sound is low, long, and gruff, but does not occur repeatedly.

1) Eructation with sour and fetid odour generally signifies a sthenic, heat syndrome, and is often caused by the retention of food or dyspepsia.

2) Eructation with sonorous sound but no putrid odour is usually due to the hyperactivity of Liver Energy which invades Stomach.

3) Frequent, odourless eructation with low sound is usually caused by the debility of Spleen-Stomach.

II. *Smelling*

1. Odour of the patient

1) Odour from the mouth

① Foul odour indicates Stomach Heat, dental caries, or oral dirtiness.

② Sour and putrid odour is generally due to the retention of food in Stomach.

③ Stinking odour as that of rotten fish signifies pulmonary abscess.

④ Fetid odour generally signifies abscess of internal organs.

2) Odour of respiration

Smell of fish or mutton is usually due to the fumigating and steaming effect of Wind-wetness-Heat.

3) Odour from the nose

Stinking odour from the nose with incessant turbid discharge indicates nasal sinusitis.

4) Odour of the body

Stinky odour of the body indicates the existence of ulcerated, malignant boil.

2. Odour of the excreta

1) Sour and fetid odour generally signifies a sthenic, heat syndrome. For example, sour and fetid stool signifies Intestinal Heat.

2) Foul and turbid urine generally signifies the downward flow of Wetness-Heat.

3) Fishy smell of excreta generally signifies an asthenic, cold syndrome, such as the debility of Spleen-Kidney Yang.

4) Leucorrhea with a slight fishy smell generally signifies the downward flow of Cold-Wetness.

Abnormal odour of patients' excreta may be found out through interrogation.

3. Odour of the ward

In critical stage, the ward may be full of bad odour.

1) Putrid odour comes from corrupted internal organs.

2) Sanguinary odour is due to the loss of blood.

3) A foul smell like that of ammonia signifies serious hydropsy (nephritis).

4) An odour of rotten apples is often encountered when the patient is suffering from diabetes mellitus.

Section 3. Interrogation

Ancient Chinese doctors had proposed that ten questions should be put to the patient, his (her) parents, relatives, or nursing personnel. They are: ① Cold and heat (chill or fever); ② Perspiration; ③ The head and body; ④ Urination and defecation; ⑤ Diet and taste; ⑥ The chest; ⑦ Sleep and hearing; ⑧ Thirst; ⑨ Anamnesis; ⑩ Cause of the disease.

Moreover, menstrual cycle and the state of menses should be inquired in females; eruptions such as smallpox, measles, etc. should be inquired in children.

Interrogation should be carried out kindly, patiently, and conscientiously. Doctors should enjoy the trust of patients in order to gain a clear idea of their situation. Now, merits of interrogation in current medicine have been incorporated in TCM, and some new styles or forms for history record have been designed on probation. But in this section, only features of TCM interrogation are discussed.

I. *Cold and heat*

Cold may be classified as aversion to cold and intolerance of cold. Heat may be classified as high fever, tidal fever, and protracted low fever, etc.

Aversion to cold indicates a chilly sensation which cannot be relieved by warming or by wearing additional clothes or quilts. It is generally a sthenic syndrome caused by an attack of exogenic Cold. Intolerance of cold can be relieved by warming or by wearing additional clothes or quilts. It is generally an asthenic syndrome caused by internal damage resulting in Yang debility.

High fever indicates the body temperature is elevated extraordinarily. It signifies a sthenic syndrome. Low fever generally occurs in the afternoon. It signifies an asthenic syndrome.

Four types of Cold and Heat are often encountered clinically.

1. Aversion to cold and elevation of body temperature

This generally belongs to the exterior syndrome which is usually classified as:

1) Exterior cold syndrome: Serious aversion to cold and mild pyrexia.

2) Exterior heat syndrome: Serious pyrexia and mild aversion to cold.

3) Attack of Wind on Taiyang: Mild pyrexia, aversion to Wind, and spontaneous perspiration.

2. Intolerance of cold without pyrexia

This generally belongs to the interior cold syndrome which is usually classified as:

1) Intolerance of cold due to internal damage, protracted illness, or the debility of Yang. This is generally an asthenic syndrome.

2) Intolerance of cold due to an attack of Cold on internal organs, such as Stomach, Intestine, etc. This is generally a sthenic

syndrome.

3. Only Heat, without Cold

These are commonly encountered in an interior heat syndrome.

1) High fever

Generally, the body temperature is higher than 39°C; instead of aversion to cold, there is aversion to heat, accompanied with flushing, thirst, longing for cold drinks, abundant perspiration, and full and large pulse. This may be caused by the wrestling of Healthy Energy with pathogenic evils, or *an excess of Yang brings about Heat.*

2) Tidal fever

Generally, it occours or is aggravated in the afternoon.

① Hectic fever due to the deficiency of Yin: It is accompanied with flushing of the zygomatic region and night sweat.

② Tidal fever due to Wetness-Warm: The patient's body is not very hot on palpation, but it becomes scorchingly hot after a while. The fever is prominent in the afternoon, accompanied with a sensation of heaviness of the head and body, and oppression in the chest. There is greasy coating of the tongue, etc.

③ Tidal fever of Yangming: The body temperature is comparatively higher in the afternoon, especially at the sunset, accompanied with abdominal distension and constipation, etc.

3) Protracted low fever

① Low fever due to the deficiency of Yin or Blood.

② Low fever due to the deficiency of Vital Energy.

Under certain circumstances, the deficiency of Vital Energy may also result in high fever, accompanied with shortness of breath, spontaneous perspiration, feebleness, etc.

4. Alternate spells of Cold and Heat

1) Half-exterior and half-interior syndrome of Shaoyang

This is characterized by an irregular onset of alternate Cold and Heat, accompanied with bitter taste, dry throat, dizziness, feeling of fullness and discomfort in the chest and hypochondria.

2) Malaria

This is characterized by shivering with cold at first, thereby ardent fever. Such onset may occur at regular time everyday, every other day, or every third day, accompanied with serious headache, thirst, hyperhidrosis, etc. After onset, the patient is as normal as usual.

II. *Perspiration*

Both exopathic attack and internal damage may cause abnormal sweating, such as hyperhidrosis, anhidrosis, etc.

1. Exterior syndrome differentiated according to the state of perspiration

1) When there are serious aversion to cold, mild fever, rigidity of the neck and nape, headache, and floating, tense pulse without perspiration, it signifies a sthenic exterior syndrome.

2) When there are fever, aversion to wind, and floating, relaxed pulse with perspiration, it signifies an asthenic exterior syndrome.

3) When there are high fever, slight aversion to cold, headache, sore throat, and floating, rapid pulse with perspiration, it signifies an asthenic, exterior, heat syndrome.

2. Interior syndrome differentiated according to the state of perspiration

1) Spontaneous perspiration

The patient perspires spontaneously by day, especially during physical labour. There are also intolerance of cold, listlessness, feebleness, etc. Generally, this signifies a deficiency of Defence Yang.

2) Night sweat

The patient does not perspire by day or when he (she) is awake. This is often accompanied with tidal fever, flushing of the zygomatic region, etc., and signifies an Yin deficiency.

3) Profuse perspiration

This may be classified as the sthenic and the asthenic.

① Steaming, incessant perspiration accompanied with flushing, thirst, longing for cold drinks, full and large pulse, etc., signifies a sthenic heat syndrome. It may be caused by an invasion of exopathic evil which transforms into Heat, or by an inward transmission of exogenic Wind-Heat.

② Cold, dripping sweat, pale complexion, cold limbs, apathy and faint pulse signify the exhaustion or collapse of Yang.

3. Differentiation of local perspiration

1) Perspiration on the forehead

This is generally caused by Heat in Upper Energizer, upward steaming of Wetness-Heat in Middle Energizer, or upward escaping of Yang in a critical condition.

2) Hemihidrosis

This indicates sweating on the left, right, upper, or lower half of the body, while the other half remains adiaphoretic. It is commonly seen in patients suffering from apoplexy, paraplegia, etc.

3) Perspiration at palms and soles

Generally, such perspiration is more evident from afternoon to night. It is usually caused by the deficiency of Yin or Wetness-Heat in Middle Energizer.

III. *The head and body*

1. Headache

1) Differentiation of headache according to various causes

① Headache due to exopathic attack: This is characterized by acute onset, serious and sustained aching, and may be classified as the following three types:

Headache due to Wind-Cold: The headache involves the nape and is aggravated when the patient comes across wind and cold. There are pyrexia and aversion to cold concurrently.

Headache due to Wind-Heat: The headache is distending as if it will split and is aggravated when the patient comes across wind and heat. There are aversion to heat and pyrexia concurrently.

Headache due to Wind-Wetness: The headache is accompanied with feeling of heaviness of the head as if it is wrapped, feeling of heaviness and weariness of the body and limbs, and feeling of oppression in the chest. There is also anorexia.

② Headache due to internal damage: This is characterized by slow onset, and moderate aching now and then. It may be classified as the following six types:

Headache due to the deficiency of Vital Energy: The headache is continuous and is accompanied with dizziness, feebleness, spontaneous perspiration, weak pulse, etc. Symptoms and signs are aggravated during physical labour.

Headache due to the deficiency of Blood: The headache is aggravated in the afternoon and accompanied with palpitation, dizziness, pale complexion and lips, even vexation and feeling of hotness at palms and soles. The pulse may be thready and weak, or thready and rapid.

Headache due to Kidney Asthenia: The headache is accompanied with a feeling of emptiness, and there are soreness and weakness of the waist and knees.

Headache due to the hyperactivity of Liver Yang: There is a feeling of distension and dizziness concurrently. Symptoms are aggravated during anger. Vexation, insomnia, stringy pulse, etc., are often encountered.

Headache due to Phlegm-Wetness: The headache is distending, accompanied with dizziness and heaviness as if the head is wrapped. Gastric oppression and nausea may occur simultaneously.

Headache due to Blood stasis: This indicates a protracted or stabbing pain at a fixed locale of the head, which is often accompanied with a history of traumatic injury.

2) Differentiation of headache according to the theory of Meridians

① Headache of Taiyang occurs at the occipital part, involving the nape.

② Headache of Yangming occurs at the forehead, involving the supraorbital bone.

③ Headache of Shaoyang occurs on both sides of the head, involving the ears.

④ Headache of Jueyin occurs at the top of the head; both eyes may be involved.

⑤ Headache of Shaoyin involves the teeth. Generally it is aggravated at night and alleviated by day.

3) Migraine

Migraine is a special kind of headache which breaks out suddenly with a lancinating nature. After an onset, the patient resumes his (her) normal state. It is generally caused by Wind-Fire in Liver or Gallbladder.

2. Vertigo

Vertigo is a disordered state in which the patient feels as if he (she) is sitting in a rocking boat, or as if the sky and earth is spinning round, thereby the patient cannot stand up. It is often accompanied with nausea and vomit, and may be either sthenic or asthenic.

1) Vertigo and distending headache

This is generally caused by the upward hyperactivity of Liver Yang, aggravated during anger, and accompanied with flushing, tinnitus, bitter taste, and irascibility.

2) Vertigo and sleepiness

This is generally caused by the internal obstruction of Phlegm-Wetness, and often accompanied with feeling of oppression in the chest, anorexia, nausea, and vomit.

3) Vertigo and dim eyesight

This is generally caused by the deficiency of both Vital Energy and Blood, and aggravated after over-exertion. It is often accompanied with pale complexion, listlessness, feebleness, and palpitation.

4) Vertigo and tinnitus

This is generally caused by the depletion of Kidney Essence or Marrow Sea, and often accompanied with pollution, amnesia, soreness and weakness of the waist and knees.

3. The body

1) Pantalgia and feeling of bodily heaviness

① Pantalgia: Pantalgia is commonly encountered in an exopathic attack of Wind-Cold, or Wind-Wetness, due to the impeded flow of Vital Energy and Blood.

Serious pantalgia as if the patient is flogged by a stick, accompanied with flushing and skin eruption, signifies an epidemic virulent Summer-Heat and Wetness.

Pantalgia in a bedridden patient indicates the impairment of Vital Energy Flow due to protracted lying.

② Feeling of bodily heaviness: Feeling of bodily heaviness accompanied with feeling of oppression in the chest, anorexia, loose stool, and greasy coating of the tongue, signifies an invasion of Wetness.

Feeling of bodily heaviness accompanied with lassitude, laziness in talking, shortness of breath, signifies the deficiency of Spleen Energy.

2) Arthralgia

Arthralgia is generally caused by Wind-Cold-Wetness mixedly, and may be classified as:

① Arthralgia principally caused by Wind: This is characterized by its migratory nature.

② Arthralgia principally caused by Cold: This is characterized by serious pain which can be alleviated by warming and is aggravated when being cooled.

③ Arthralgia principally caused by Wetness: This is characterized by fixed pain and feeling of heaviness.

④ Arthralgia of the heat type: There are redness, hotness, swelling, and pain of joints which signify the exogenic Wind-Cold-Wetness have been transformed into Heat.

3) Lumbago

① Vague pain and weakness of the waist which are aggravated in the afternoon, signify Kidney Asthenia.

② Cold pain and feeling of heaviness of the waist which are aggravated during overcast or rainy days, signify an attack of Cold-Wetness.

③ Hot pain, feeling of distension and heaviness of the waist, accompanied with frequent micturition, urodynia, and deep-coloured urine, signify the downward flow of Wetness-Heat.

④ Fixed, stabbing pain of the waist which is unable to bend over or turn round, may be caused by injury from falls, contusions, or strains.

⑤ Sudden onset of serious pain at the waist, accompanied with hematuria, generally indicate stranguria caused by the passage of urinary stone.

IV. *The chest, hypochondria, epigastrium, and abdomen*

1. The chest

Symptoms and signs of the chest are generally due to disorders of Lung and Heart.

1) Feeling of oppression in the chest, palpitation, shortness of breath, spontaneous perspiration, and weak or irregular pulse generally signify the insufficiency of Heart Energy.

2) On the basis of Heart Energy insufficiency, if there are cold limbs and aversion to cold, it signifies an insufficiency of Heart Yang.

3) Dizziness, pallor, palpitation, dysphoria, insomnia, and thready, weak pulse signify the deficiency of Heart Blood.

4) Palpitation, dysphoria, insomnia, amnesia or even night sweat, low fever, dry mouth, reddened tongue with little saliva, and faint or rapid pulse signify the deficiency of Heart Yin.

5) Serious chest pain radiating to the back, palpitation, accompanied with cyanosis, cold limbs, stabbing or oppressive pain at the precordial region signify a true Heart pain, caused by a sudden obstruction of Heart Collaterals.

6) Shortness of breath, low and weak voice, aversion to wind, spontaneous perspiration, and pale complexion suggest the insufficiency of Lung Energy.

7) Feeling of chest stuffiness, shortness of breath, fever, cough, dyspnea, even nausea suggest the stagnation of Lung Energy.

8) Cough, emaciation, hectic fever, night sweat, lassitude, and expectoration of blood-tinged phlegm suggest a consumptive disease.

9) Fever, chest pain, expectoration of pus and blood with an offensive smell of rotten fish suggest pulmonary abscess.

10) Ardent fever, dyspnea, flaring of nares, and expectoration of rusty sputum suggest an exuberance of Lung Heat.

2. The hypochondria

Symptoms and signs of the hypochondria are generally caused by disorders of Liver and Gallbladder.

1) Dizziness, headache, flushing, tinnitus, deafness, fullness and pain of the chest and hypochondrium, belching, acid regurgitation, and stringy and energetic pulse suggest an upward invasion of hyperactive Liver Energy.

2) Wandering, distending pain at the hypochondriac region, feeling of oppression in the chest, accompanied with heaving sighs and irascibility, are generally due to the depression or stagnation of Liver Energy.

3) Bitter taste in the mouth, dry throat, dysphoria, restlessness, feeling of fullness in the chest and hypochondria, dizziness, congested eyes, irritability, redness of lateral sides of the tongue with yellow coating, stringy and rapid pulse signify Liver Heat.

4) Jaundice and distending pain at the hypochondria, accompanied with anorexia, nausea, and deep-coloured urine, are generally due to the accumulation and stagnation of Wetness-Heat in Liver-Gallbladder.

5) Feeling of fullness and discomfort in the chest and hypochondria, alternate spells of fever and chill, easiness to be frightened while lying on the side, and constipation with dry stool suggest the accumulation of virulent Heat in Liver or Liver abscess.

3. The epigastrium

1) Sudden onset of epigastric cold pain which may be alleviated by warming, indicates an attack of Cold on Stomach.

2) Feeling of fullness and distending pain at the epigastric region, involving both hypochondria, which are aggravated during anger and alleviated after eructation, signifies the stagnation of Stomach Energy caused by the transverse invasion of depressed Liver.

3) Burning pain at the epigastric region, gastric discomfort with acid regurgitation, halitosis, constipation, yet polyphagia, signify the flaming up of Stomach Fire.

4) Vague gastralgia which becomes evident when the stomach is empty, desire for being pressed and warmed, nausea, watery vomitus, are manifestations of Asthenia and Cold of Stomach.

5) Burning pain at the epigastric region, gastric discomfort with acid regurgitation, anorexia, dry mouth, constipation, vexation, hotness at palms and soles, reddened tongue, thready and rapid pulse, signify the depletion of Stomach Yin and the existence of asthenic Fire.

6) Fixed, stabbing pain at the epigastric region, purplish black vomitus, and/or tarry stool, signify Blood stasis in gastric Collaterals.

7) Feeling of stuffiness and distending pain in the stomach, eructation with putrid odour, acid regurgitation, and alleviation of symptoms after vomit, suggest food retention in the stomach.

4. The abdomen

1) Abdominal distension, cold and pain in the epigastrium, anorexia, loose stools, cold limbs, pale tongue with white coating, feeble and slow pulse, signify a cold syndrome caused by the debility of Spleen Yang.

2) Anorexia, abdominal distension after meal, dizziness, lassitude, chronic diarrhea, suggest the deficiency of Spleen-Stomach Energy.

3) Intermittent abdominal colic and abdominal mass which may be dispersed or shifted by pressing, or even vomiting of ascaris, suggest a parasitic infestation.

4) Distending pain of the lower abdomen, accompanied with difficulty in micturition, suggest uroschesis.

5) Abdominal pain and tenderness of the lower abdomen on the right side, accompanied with pyrexia, anorexia, and abdominal distension, suggest periappendicular abscess.

V. *The ear and the eye*

1. The ear

1) Tinnitus

Tinnitus is a sensation of noise like the shrilling sound of cicada. It may occur on one side or on both sides, intermittently or continuously.

① Sudden onset of loud tinnitus, which is aggravated when the ear is pressed, or which is serious by day and becomes mitigated at night, generally signifies a sthenic syndrome caused by the upward harassment of Liver-Gallbladder Fire.

② Gradual onset of low tinnitus, which is alleviated when the ear is pressed, or which becomes mitigated by day and serious at night, generally signifies an asthenic syndrome caused by the depletion of Kidney Energy.

2) Hypoacusis

① Sudden onset of hypoacusis accompanied with a stifled sensation and/or headache is generally due to the obstruction of hearing by Wind-Fire, or Liver Fire.

② Gradual onset of hypoacusis accompanied with soreness and weakness of the waist and knees is generally due to the deficiency of Kidney Yin.

3) Deafness

① Sudden onset of deafness accompanied with alternate spells of chills and fever, bitter taste, dry throat, dizziness, etc., is due to an Attack of Cold on Shaoyang.

② Gradual onset of deafness in protracted illness or old patients generally signifies the exhaustion of Primordial Energy.

2. The eye

1) Ophthalmalgia

① Serious ophthalmalgia involving the head and accompanied with nausea and vomit, mydriasis, and opacity of lens, signifies an internal oculopathy caused by various kinds of Wind.

② Stabbing ophthalmalgia, spasm of ocular connector accompanied with headache and dizziness, signify an upward assault of virulent Fire from Heart Meridian.

③ Swelling and pain of the eye, conjunctival congestion, photophobia, and aversion to wind are manifestations of epidemic conjunctivitis.

④ Photophobia of both eyes without pain and fever generally signifies the deficiency of Blood.

2) Dizziness

① Dizziness accompanied with tinnitus, soreness and weakness of the waist and knees, generally signifies the upward hyperactivity of Liver Yang on the basis of Kidney Yin deficiency.

② Dizziness accompanied with feeling of oppression in the chest, nausea, and vomit, generally signifies an internal obstruction of Phlegm-Wetness.

3) Dysopia

Blurred vision and xerophthalmia are manifestations of the depletion of Vital Energy and Blood.

4) Nyctalopia is generally caused by Liver Asthenia.

VI. *Diet and taste*

1. Dipsia and water intake

Whether the patient is thirsty or not, and how much water the patient drinks, reflect the vicissitude of his (her) body fluids. These serve as indices by which Cold or Heat, Asthenia or Sthenia may be differentiated.

1) Adipsia

This indicates that the patient is not thirsty, or thirsty but only longing for a small amount of hot drink. Such states signify a cold syndrome or the body fluids have not been damaged.

2) Polydipsia

Polydipsia signifies a serious depletion of body fluids.

① Dire thirst and longing for a large quantity of cold drink, accompanied with fever, perspiration, etc., indicate a sthenic, heat syndrome.

② Polydipsia accompanied with polyuria, polyphagia, and emaciation, indicates diabetes mellitus.

③ Polydipsia may occur after excessive perspiration, violent vomit or diarrhea, or intense diuretic therapy.

3) Thirst without longing for much drink

① Dry mouth, tidal fever, night sweat, but no desire to drink signify a deficiency of Yin.

② Thirst with scanty water intake, recessive fever, feeling of heaviness and weariness of the body generally signify the obstruction of Vital Energy flow caused by Wetness-Heat.

③ Thirst, desire for hot water but the intake is not much, or accompanied with watery vomitus and dizziness, generally signify an internal retention of Phlegm-Fluid.

④ Dry mouth, desire for gargling water but showing reluctance to swallow it, dim cyanotic tongue, etc., signify the existence of Blood stasis.

2. Appetite and food intake

1) Anorexia

① Anorexia, emaciation, abdominal distension, loose stool, feebleness, and weak pulse signify an asthenic syndrome.

② Anorexia with feeling of oppression in the stomach and heaviness of the body and limbs, greasy coating of the tongue signify the existense of Wetness or the debility of Spleen Yang.

③ Anorexia and repugnance to oily food, accompanied with jaundice, hypochondriac pain, nausea, vomit, etc., signify the accumulation and stagnation of Wetness-Heat in Liver-Gallbladder.

④ Food repugnance accompanied with epigastric fullness and distension, eructation with putrid and sour odour, etc., generally suggest food retention due to overeating.

⑤ Aversion to food odour or vomit right after eating in females is commonly a sign of pregnancy.

2) Hyperorexia

① Hyperorexia accompanied with thirst, halitosis, constipation, and vexation, etc., signifies the exuberance of Stomach Fire.

② Polyorexia accompanied with loose stool signifies Stomach is strong while Spleen is weak.

③ A sudden spurt of appetite prior to collapse signifies the impending exhaustion of Spleen-Stomach Energy.

3) Hunger but with a poor appetite

This is commonly accompanied with gastric discomfort, acid regurgitation, pyrosis, and thready, rapid pulse. These signify the existence of Stomach Yin deficiency complicated by asthenic Fire.

4) Pica

① Predilection for clay, raw rice, etc., accompanied with abdominal distension and pain, emaciation, and periumbilical mass in children, generally signify a parasitic infestation.

② Predilection for sour fruits, vinegar, etc., accompanied with nausea, menolipsis in married women, generally signifies pregnancy.

3. Gustatory sensation in the mouth and odours from it

1) Tastelessness accompanied with poor appetite generally signifies the deficiency of Spleen-Stomach Energy.

2) Sweet taste or stickiness within the mouth, accompanied with feeling of heaviness and weariness of the body, thick and greasy coating of the tongue, generally signifies the existence of Phlegm-Wetness.

3) Bitter taste generally signifies Stomach Heat or Gallbladder Heat.

4) Sour and putrid odour from the mouth indicates dyspepsia due to improper eating.

5) Salty taste signifies Kidney Asthenia.

6) Halitosis is due to the exuberance of Stomach Fire.

VII. *Sleep*

According to TCM, insomnia is due to the failure of Yang to be admitted into Yin, while lethargy is due to the failure of Yang to depart from Yin.

1. Insomnia

Insomnia may be classified as difficulty in falling asleep, unsound sleep, easiness to be aroused, lying awake all night, etc.

1) Difficulty in falling asleep accompanied with vexation and hotness of palms and soles, soreness and weakness of the waist and knees, is generally due to the breakdown of normal physiological

coordination between Heart and Kidney.

2) Easiness to be aroused accompanied with palpitation, amnesia, anorexia, and feebleness, is generally caused by the debility of both Heart and Spleen and/or Blood deficiency.

3) Insomnia accompanied with feeling of fullness, distension, and oppression in the epigastric region, eructation with putrid and sour odour, thick and greasy coating of the tongue, is generally caused by food retention in the stomach. *Disorders of Stomach results in restless sleep.*

4) Insomnia accompanied with dyspnea, palpitation, hydropsy, etc., is generally due to the debility of Heart-Kidney Yang.

2. Drowsiness or lethargy

1) Drowsiness accompanied with feeling of oppression in the chest, heaviness and weariness of the body, greasy coating of the tongue, and soft pulse, signify the debility of Spleen Yang and the exuberance of Wetness, thereby the uprising of Lucid Yang is impeded.

2) Drowsiness after meal, accompanied with shortness of breath, feebleness, deep and weak pulse, is generally due to Spleen Asthenia.

3) Lethargy accompanied with fever which becomes serious at night, crimson tongue, and rapid pulse, signify an attack of Pericardium by Heat.

VIII. *Defecation and urination*

1. Defecation

1) Constipation

This indicates delayed defecation or dyschesia with dry or hardened stool.

① Heat constipation: Constipation accompanied with fever, fullness and distension of the abdomen, halitosis, as well as reddened tongue with yellow and dry coating, is due to the depletion of body fluids by exuberant Heat.

② Cold constipation: Constipation accompanied with pale complexion, intolerance of cold, longing for hot drinks, deep and slow pulse, is often encountered in old people, caused by the debility of Yang.

③ Asthenic constipation: Constipation accompanied with manifestations of the deficiency of Vital Energy or Blood is commonly seen in patients suffering from protracted illness or in postpartum women.

④ Constipation due to the depression and stagnation of Liver Energy: This kind of constipation is accompanied with feeling of fullness and distension in the hypochondria, irascibility, stringy and thready pulse.

2) Diarrhea

This indicates abnormally frequent intestinal evacuations with loose or watery stools. Sometimes there are undigested cereals mixed in the stool.

① Asthenic cold diarrhea: This is characterized by abdominal pain before diarrhea or diarrhea before dawn, loose or watery stool mixed with undigested cereals, anorexia, abdominal distension, cold and soreness of the waist and knees.

② Wetness-Heat diarrhea: This is characterized by yellow, sticky, and foul stool, burning heat sensation at the anus during defecation, frequent defecation with scanty feces, abdominal pain or tenesmus. Wetness-Heat diarrhea with tenesmus is a feature of dysentery.

③ Diarrhea due to improper eating: This is characterized by feeling of fullness and oppression in the epigastric region, eructation with putrid odour, undigested cereals in stools, and the abdominal pain is alleviated after defecation.

④ Diarrhea due to the depression and stagnation of Liver Energy: This signifies Spleen is attacked by hyperactive Liver. Diarrhea occurs during emotional depression and the abdominal pain is alleviated after defecation.

2. Urination

The vicissitude of body fluids and the functional states of Lung, Spleen, and Kidney may be inferred from the amount of urine and the frequency of micturition, etc.

1) Abnormal variations in the amount of urine

① Increased amount of urine: Abundant, clear urine, especially at night, intolerance of cold, are manifestations of an asthenic cold syndrome, generally caused by the debility of Kidney Yang.

② Decreased amount of urine: Scanty, deep-coloured urine generally signifies a heat syndrome or the consumption of body fluids caused by excessive sweating, vomit, or diarrhea.

In hydropsy, oliguria is usually caused by the dysfunction of Lung, Spleen, and Kidney.

2) Abnormal variations in the frequency of micturition

① Frequent, hard-going urodynia and urgency of micturition, accompanied with deep-coloured scanty urine, signify a Wetness-Heat syndrome in Lower Energizer.

② Frequent micturition with clear urine or increased nocturnal urine discharge suggests Kidney Asthenia.

③ Enuresis indicates an involuntary urine discharge during sleep. It occurs often in children due to the immaturity of Visceral function.

④ Failure to stop micturition immediately after discharge is commonly seen in the aged due to the unconsolidation of Kidney Energy.

⑤ Incontinence of urine indicates failure to initiate and stop micturition, dripping of urine day and night. This is generally due to the unconsolidation of Kidney Energy and the loss of restraint of Urinary Bladder.

⑥ Hard-going urination, urodynia, urgency of micturition with burning sensation during discharge suggest stranguria.

IX. *Menstruation, leucorrhea, pregnancy, and child-bearing*

1. Menstruation

Normal menstruation begins at 13～15 years of age in females with a period of 28 days approximately and a duration of 3～5 days. Generally, it stops around 49 years of age according to TCM. But there are physiological variations, such as bimonthly menses, seasonal menses, or even annual menses. Some women do not menstruate all their lives, yet they may be pregnant. During pregnancy and lactation, generally menstruation does not occur.

1) Menstrual cycle

① Preceded menstrual cycle: This indicates the menstruation is preceded for more than 8～9 days.

Abundant, deep red, sticky menses signifies Blood Heat.

Abundant, light red, dilute menses signifies Asthenia of Vital Energy.

Purplish red menses accompanied with feeling of distension and pain in hypochondria and breasts, signifies the harassment of Liver Energy.

② Delayed menstrual cycle: This indicates the menstruation is delayed for more than 8～9 days.

Scanty, light red, dilute menses signifies Blood deficiency.

Scanty, dim purple menses with clots signifies Blood stasis caused by Cold.

Purplish red menses with clots and distending pain of the lower abdomen signifies the stagnation of Vital Energy.

③ Irregular menstrual cycle: This indicates the deviation is more than 8～9 days.

Scanty, purplish red menses with clots and distending pain of breasts signifies the depression of Liver Energy.

Light red, dilute menses with variable quantities signifies the debility of Spleen-Kidney.

2) Menstrual quantity

Usually it amounts to 50～100 ml.

① Menorrhagia: This indicates an increased amount of menses and a prolonged duration of menstruation.

Menorrhagia with purplish red and sticky menses signifies Blood Heat.

Menorrhagia with light red and dilute menses signifies the deficiency of Vital Energy.

② Hypomenorrhea: This indicates scanty menses and shortened duration of menstruation, and may be caused by the deficiency of Blood, or the stagnation of Blood flow due to the impediment of Cold or Phlegm-Wetness.

③ Metrorrhagia and *leaking menstruation*: Metrorrhagia indicates a sudden onset of excessive menorrhagia which fails to stop; *leaking menstruation* indicates menses dripping incessantly. Generally, they are caused by the debility of Vital and Conception Vessel Meridians and may be differentiated as various types: Vital Energy deficiency, Blood Heat, Blood stasis, etc.

3) Colour and quality of menses

Under normal circumstances, the menses is red in colour, neither dilute nor curdy.

Light red and dilute menses, even like water in which meat has been washed, signifies the deficiency of both Vital Energy and Blood.

Deep red and sticky menses generally signifies an exuberance of Blood Heat.

Dim purple menses with clots and lower abdominal pain signifies a cold syndrome or the existence of Blood stasis.

4) Dysmenorrhea

This indicates lower abdominal pain occurring cyclically around menstruation.

Distending lower abdominal pain which occurs before or during menstruation and disappears after menstruation, signifies a sthenic syndrome. This is generally caused by Vital Energy stagnation and Blood stasis.

Continuous vague lower abdominal pain after menstruation, accompanied with soreness of the waist, signifies an asthenic syndrome. This is generally caused by the debility of Kidney.

Lower abdominal pain during menstruation which may be relieved by warming, signifies a cold syndrome.

2. Morbid leucorrhea

Normally, there is a small amount of milky white secretion in the vagina which is odourless. Variations in its quantity, colour, odour, and quality indicate a morbid state.

1) Leucorrhea

Abundant, dilute, dripping vaginal discharge without offensive odour signifies a cold-wetness syndrome, which may be caused by Spleen Asthenia, or the downward flow of Cold-Wetness.

2) Yellowish vaginal discharge

Abundant, yellowish, sticky vaginal discharge with fetid odour signifies a Wetness-Heat syndrome, or a downward flow of Wetness-Heat.

3) Leucorrhea with bloody discharge

Reddish, odourless, sticky leucorrhea or leucorrhea mixed with blood generally signifies the injury of Uterine Collaterals, such as caused by Heat transformed from the depression of Liver Energy.

Moreover, continuous dripping leucorrhea after menopause suggests cancerization and should be examined meticulously.

3. Pregnancy

Sudden menolipsis of a married woman with slippery pulse but no evident symptoms and signs suggests an early pregnancy.

1) Morning sickness or pernicious vomiting

This indicates nausea, repeated vomit, and inability to take food because of pregnancy.

① Morning sickness accompanied with listlessness, lassitude, tastelessness, and abdominal distension, signifies the weakness of Spleen-Stomach and the upward offending of Fetal Energy.

② Morning sickness accompanied with emotional depression, irascibility, bitter taste, and acid regurgitation, signifies the exuberance of Liver Fire which attacks Stomach.

③ Morning sickness accompanied with feeling of oppression in the chest, anorexia, vomit of sputum and saliva, signifies the adverse uprising of Phlegm-Turbidity.

2) Threatened abortion

This indicates bearing-down pain of the waist and abdomen, bleeding from the vagina, and continuous moving of the fetus.

① Threatened abortion accompanied with dim complexion, dizziness, tinnitus, soreness and weakness of the waist and knees, and frequent micturition, signifies the deficiency of Kidney Energy and the debility of Vital and Conception Vessel Meridians.

② Threatened abortion accompanied with pale complexion, listlessness, lassitude, etc., signifies the debility of Spleen and the deficiency of Blood.

Moreover, falling, dodging, or contusion may also cause abdominal pain and vaginal bleeding in pregnant women.

4. Postpartum condition

1) Persisted lochiorrhea

This indicates a persistent vaginal discharge over 20 days after child-birth.

① Abundant, pale-coloured, dilute lochiorrhea accompanied with sallow complexion, listlessness, and feebleness, signifies the sinking of Spleen Energy due to its Asthenia.

② Reddish, sticky lochiorrhea accompanied with flushing, thirst, constipation, and deep coloured urine, signifies Blood Heat.

③ Dim purple lochiorrhea with clots accompanied by stabbing pain in the lower abdomen which is resistant to pressing, signifies Blood stasis.

2) Postpartum fever

① Fever with chills, accompanied by aching of the head and body, is generally due to an exogenic attack of Cold.

② High fever, fretfulness, thirst, longing for cold drinks, constipation, and deep-coloured urine signifies an exuberance of Heat or Fire.

③ Continuous low fever, abdominal pain, dizziness, blurred vision, constipation with dry and hard stool signify Blood deficiency and the resultant asthenic Heat.

X. *Children*

Inquiry of children about their illness is usually difficult. Therefore, their parents, relatives, or nurses are interrogated.

1. Prenatal condition

In examining a newborn, we should inquire of its mother about the nutritional state during her pregnancy and problems encountered in her delivery and lactation, to assess the level of its congenital endowment.

2. Postnatal condition

This includes the development of its sitting, crawling, standing, walking, dentition, speaking, and the state of its feeding.

3. History of prophylactic vaccination

History of prophylactic vaccination, and infectious diseases suffered from or contacted with, should be interrogated.

4. Probable causes of the current disease

These should be put forward to its parents or nurses.

Since children are tender and weak, and their defence mechanism has not been fully consolidated, they are apt to suffer from infectious diseases, dyspepsia, etc.

Other aspects which had not been included in Ten Questions cited above, but were also put forward clinically by ancient Chinese doctors are similar to those in current medicine. They are anamnesis, family history, and life style.

XI. *Anamnesis*

A newly suffered disease is generally sthenic; a chronic disease is generally asthenic; a recurrent disease is generally asthenic, complicated by sthenic syndromes.

One who usually suffers from an upward hyperactivity of Liver Yang, is apt to have a stroke. One who usually suffers from diarrhea is usually asthenic in Spleen Yang. Manic-depressive psychosis is often triggered by emotional agitation.

The course of treatment and the appropriateness or inappropriateness of drugs administered contribute greatly to the management of the present illness. For example, if no satisfactory therapeutic effect has been obtained by the administration of cool-or cold-natured drugs in treating a heat syndrome, there may be inadequacy of the dosage, improper compatibility of drugs in the prescription, or a mistake in syndrome differentiation. If the disease condition is aggravated or new symptoms and signs occur after medication, the cause or causes should be investigated.

XII. *Family history*

This contributes to the discovery of certain hereditary or congenital diseases, or an infectious disease, such as tuberculosis, syphilis, etc.

XIII. *Life style*

This includes the patient's dietary habits and predilections, occupation, frame of mind, economic state, life experience, etc., which may be related to the present illness.

Section 4. Pulse Feeling and Palpation

I. *Pulse feeling*

    1. Significance of pulse feeling

Pulse feeling is an important diagnostic method in TCM. The vicissitude of pathogenic evils and Healthy Energy may be detected through pulse feeling and a certain type of pulse indicates a particular syndrome generally.

    2. Locale for pulse feeling

In ancient China, pulse feeling was carried out at various parts of the body. With the passage of time, only radial artery at the wrist is felt by Traditional Chinese doctors.

Pulse feeling on radial artery at the wrist as an independent diagnostic method begins in the third century (Jin Dynasty) when Wang Shuhe published his *The Pulse Classics*. According to Wang Shuhe, the radial artery at the wrist is divided into three portions: Inch, Bar, and Cubit. Bar corresponds to the medial side of the styloid process of radius, while Inch is situated ahead of Bar and Cubit is situated behind Bar. Inch pulse is felt with the tip of the doctor's index finger; Bar pulse is felt with the tip of his middle finger; and Cubit pulse is felt with his ring finger.

There are six portions on both wrists, and they had been designated as follows (Fig. Assignation of Viscera to Six Portions of

Radial Arteries).

In clinical practice, Inch, Bar, and Cubit are felt simultaneously by placing these finger tips superficially, intermediately, and deeply on them; in other words, their manifestations are felt and discriminated by light touch, moderate press, and heavy press.

It must be pointed out that such designation only signifies Visceral states may be detected at corresponding portions, but it by no means indicates the state of a special internal organ can only be detected at its corresponding portion.

3. Method of pulse feeling

1) Time for pulse feeling

Daybreak is the best time for pulse feeling, because at this time the flow of Vital Energy and Blood is not influenced by physical, mental activities and food taking. Generally, pulse feeling should be carried out in a quiet environment while the patient has been tranquilizd.

2) Posture

Let the patient sit or lie supinely, stretching his (her) forearm out with palms facing upwards at the same level of his (her) heart. A small pillow is needed for padding the wrist to be felt. Feel the pulse of the right radial artery with finger tips of the left hand and the left radial artery with finger tips of the right hand. Fingers for pulse feeling should be arched and they should be separated apart at appropriate distances according to the height of the patient. In tall patients, distances should be wider; in short patients, distances should be narrower.

Pulse feeling in children may be performed by using one finger only, because their Inch-Bar-Cubit is too short.

3) Measurement of pulse frequency

In ancient times, the pulse frequency of a patient is measured by counting the number of pulses during one respiratory cycle of the doctor. It goes without saying that such method falls out of use at present.

4) Three levels of pulse feeling

① *Touching* indicates to feel the pulse lightly or superficially;

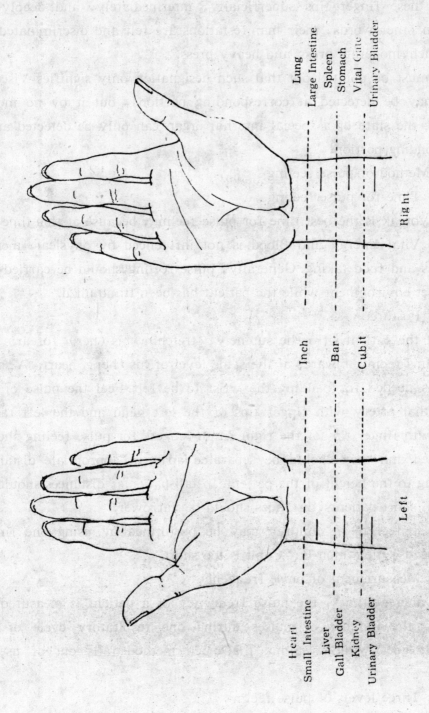

Fig. Assignation of Viscera to Six Portions of Radial Arteries

② *Searching* indicates to feel the pulse with moderate pressing;

③ *Pressing* indicates to feel the pulse with heavy pressing.

5) Duration of pulse feeling

It should not be shorter than 1 min. generally. In order to find out whether there is a *knotted* pulse, *intermittent* pulse, or *running* pulse, etc., 2 or 3 min. may be required.

4. Procedure of pulse feeling

1) Find out the locales of Inch, Bar, and Cubit, and the level of their touching, searching, and pressing.

2) Measure the pulse frequency and assess its rhythmicity.

3) Feel whether it is long or short, large or small, energetic or feeble, stringy or slippery, etc.

5. Characteristics of normal pulse

1) Normal pulse condition

A normal pulse is gentle, even, rhythmic, and energetic. It is full of Vitality, Stomach Energy, and Rootedness.

Whenever there is a sign of exertion in a feeble or faint pulse, or a sign of gentleness in a stringy or sthenic pulse, it indicates the existence of Vitality.

Whenever there is a sign of evenness in a morbid pulse, it indicates the existence of Stomach Energy.

Whenever the pulse condition of Cubit is gentle and energetic under deep and heavy pressing, it is called a *rooted* pulse which signifies the existence of Kidney Energy or Vital Gate Fire.

A pulse without Vitality, Stomach Energy, or Rootedness predicts an ominous outcome.

2) Variations of the anatomical site of radial artery

The radial artery may be ectopic. In some patients, it can only be felt at the dorsum of the wrist, or on the back of the hand.

3) Factors influencing the pulse condition

① Sex: The pulse condition in females is slightly soft, weak, and rapid. During pregnancy, their pulse condition becomes slippery.

② Age: The younger the age, the faster the pulse rate. In old people, the radial pulse becomes tough and stringy generally.

③ Constitution: Floating pulse is often felt in a lean person, deep pulse is often felt in an obese person. *Six Yin Pulse* indicates Inch-Bar-Cubit of both sides is congenitally deep and thready; *Six Yang Pulse* indicates Inch-Bar-Cubit of both sides is congenitally full and large.

④ Emotion: Emotional change may influence the pulse condition directly and immediately.

⑤ Diet: After meals, the pulse condition is generally full, slow and energetic. After prolonged hunger, the pulse condition is generally feeble. After drinking alcoholic liquor, the pulse becomes rapid and energetic.

⑥ Physical activities: After intense physical labour, the pulse becomes rapid and energetic. After rest or sleep, the pulse is slow and gentle. The pulse condition of a mental worker is generally weaker then a physical worker.

⑦ Seasonal and climatic variations: According to the theory of *correspondence between mankind and the universe*, pulse condition varies with the four seasons of a year and the change of climates. For instance, there are such accounts in *Canon of Internal Medicine*: *The pulse becomes stringy in spring, full in summer, weak and floating in autumn, stony or sinking in winter*.

6. Abnormal pulse conditions and their clinical significance

In *The Pulse Classics*, 24 kinds of abnormal pulse conditions had been described by Wang Shuhe. Along with the accumulation of clinical experience, since then 28 kinds of abnormal pulse conditions were differentiated, and they may be classified as 6 categories: the floating and the deep; the slow and the rapid; the feeble and the replete.

1) The category of floating pulse

① Floating pulse: This pulse feels distinct only on light touch and slightly weakened on pressing.

Generally, it signifies an exterior syndrome. A floating and feeble pulse signifies an exterior asthenic syndrome; a floating and energetic pulse signifies an exterior sthenic syndrome.

In a critical disease condition, the appearance of floating pulse signifies the upward escape of Yang Energy.

② Full pulse: This pulse feels full and large, coming vigorously like waves surging and going gently.

Generally, it signifies an exuberance of Vital Energy and the hyperactivity of Fire. A full and feeble pulse signifies the depletion of Yin and the soaring of exuberant Fire.

In patients suffering from protracted deficiency of Vital Energy, loss of blood, or recurrent diarrhea, the appearance of full pulse signifies a critical condition.

Note: A large pulse feels broad and it lifts the finger tip to a greater height, but without feeling of wave surging.

③ Soft pulse: This pulse feels floating, thready, and soft on light touch, but faint on heavy pressing.

Generally, it signifies an asthenic syndrome such as caused by the deficiency of Vital Energy and Blood, etc. It may also occur in a wetness syndrome.

④ Hollow pulse: This pulse feels floating, large, and hollow, like the leaf of a Chinese scallion.

Generally, it signifies a sudden, profuse loss of blood, or a critical depletion of Yin.

⑤ Tympanic pulse: This pulse feels floating, stringy, exteriorly taut and interiorly hollow, like a drum surface.

Generally, it signifies a loss of blood, such as in premature labour, metrorrhagia, or spermatorrhea.

⑥ Scattered pulse: This pulse feels floating, diffusing on light touch and faint on heavy pressing; its rhythm is irregular.

Generally, it signifies the exhaustion of Heart Energy, or the failure of Parenchymatous Viscera.

2) The category of deep pulse.

① Deep pulse: This pulse feels distinct only on heavy pressing.

Generally, it signifies an interior syndrome. A deep and feeble pulse signifies an interior asthenic syndrome; a deep and energetic pulse signifies an interior sthenic syndrome.

② Deep-sited pulse: This pulse feels deeper than the deep pulse and it can be felt only on pressing hard to the bone.

Generally, it signifies syncope, severe pain, or internal blockage due to pathogenic evils.

③ Firm pulse: This pulse feels replete, energetic, long, and slightly stringy; it can only be felt on heavy pressing.

Generally, it signifies an internal accumulation of Yin Cold, hernia, mass in the abdomen, etc.

④ Weak pulse: This pulse feels extremely soft, feeble, and thready; it can be felt only on heavy pressing.

Generally, it signifies the deficiency of Vital Energy and Blood.

3) The category of slow pulse

① Slow pulse: This indicates a pulse whose frequency is less than 60/min.

Generally, it signifies a cold syndrome. A slow and feeble pulse signifies an asthenic cold syndrome; a slow and energetic pulse signifies a sthenic cold syndrome.

② Moderate or relaxed pulse: This indicates a pulse with diminished tension and moderate frequency.

Generally, it signifies either a healthy state, or a wetness syndrome, or the debility of Spleen-Stomach. If it is a morbid state, certainly there will be other pathologic manifestations.

③ Uneven pulse: This pulse feels unsmooth while coming and going, like the scraping of bamboo with a knife.

Generally, it signifies the deficiency of Blood, Essence, or body fluids; or the stagnation of Vital Energy and Blood.

④ Knotted pulse: This indicates a pulse which is slow with irregular intervals.

Generally, it signifies the stagnation of Vital Energy and Blood.

⑤ Intermittent pulse: This pulse feels weak and slow, with pausing at regular intervals.

Generally, it signifies a disorder of Heart, or the debility of

Parenchymatous Viscera.

4) The category of rapid pulse

① Rapid pulse: This indicates a pulse whose frequency is faster than 90/min.

Generally, it signifies a heat syndrome. A rapid and feeble pulse signifies an asthenic heat syndrome; a rapid and energetic pulse signifies a sthenic heat syndrome.

② Swift pulse: This indicates a pulse whose frequency is about 120~140/min.

Generally, it signifies the hyperactivity of Yang, or the exhaustion of Yin.

③ Slippery pulse: This pulse feels slippery while it comes and goes.

Generally, it signifies a sthenic syndrome, or the existence of Phlegm, dyspepsia, as well as pregnancy.

④ Running pulse: This pulse feels hasty and rapid, with irregular intermittence.

Generally, it signifies the exuberance of sthenic Heat, the stagnation of Vital Energy and Blood, the retention of Phlegm-Fluid, or dyspepsia.

⑤ Tremulous pulse: This pulse feels slippery, rapid, and energetic, like a bouncing pea.

Generally, it signifies a state of being frightened, pain, or pregnancy.

5) The category of feeble pulse

① Feeble pulse: This pulse feels soft, feeble, and hollow.

Generally, it signifies the deficiency of Vital Energy and Blood, or the depletion of body fluids.

② Thready or Small pulse: This pulse feels thin and feeble, yet easily perceptible.

Generally, it signifies the exhaustion of Vital Energy and Blood, or other kinds of deficiency.

③ Indistinct pulse: This pulse feels extremely soft and thready, discernible at one moment, indistinct at another.

Generally, it signifies the collapse of Yang, or the extreme exhaustion of Vital Energy and Blood.

④ Short pulse: This indicates a pulse which is distinct only at Bar or of a short extent.

A short and feeble pulse signifies the deficiency of Vital Energy and/or Blood. A short and energetic pulse signifies the depression of Vital Energy, the accumulation of Phlegm, or dyspepsia.

6) The category of replete pulse

① Replete pulse: This pulse feels vigorous in coming and going, and energetic on light touch and heavy pressing too.

Generally, it signifies a sthenic syndrome.

② Stringy pulse: This pulse feels straight and long, like the string of a musical instrument.

Generally, it signifies the hyperactivity of Liver and Gallbladder, pain or the retention of Phlegm or Fluid.

③ Tense pulse: This pulse feels tense and energetic, like a cord stretched tight.

Generally, it signifies the existence of Cold, pain, or dyspepsia.

④ Long pulse: This pulse feels extending longer than Inch-Bar-Cubit.

Generally, a long and moderate pulse signifies a healthy state; a long and stiff pulse signifies both the pathogenic evil and the Healthy Energy are exuberant.

7. Summary

1) Two or more than two morbid pulse conditions may occur simultaneously, signifying a complicated pathologic situation. For instance, floating and tense pulse signifies an exterior cold syndrome; deep and rapid pulse signifies an interior heat syndrome; deep, thready, and stringy pulse signifies the deficiency of Yin and the hyperactivity of Liver, etc.

2) Generally, pulse conditions conform to symptoms and signs, but there may be exceptions, due to the extreme complexity of pathogenesis. Therefore, sometimes we make a diagnosis on the basis of symptoms and signs rather than on pulse condition; sometimes we make a diagnosis on the basis of pulse condition rather than on symptoms and signs.

3) Scientific measures and objective indices have been tried to reflect these pulse conditions confirmed by veteran Traditional Chinese doctors, as they rely mainly on subjective feelings. Nevertheless, up to now, no satisfactory results have been obtained and it remains to be a difficult task in medical research.

II. *Palpation*

Generally speaking, the method of Palpation in TCM is similar to that in current medicine. It is used to find out whether there is cold or heat, dryness or wetness, slippery or uneven, soft or hard, edema or induration, etc. Among them, the identification of whether there is tenderness at the acupoint or acupoints along specific Meridians is a feature of TCM. For instance, tenderness at Weishu (B*21*), Pishu (B*20*), and Zusanli (S*36*) suggests gastropathy; tenderness at Ganshu (B*18*), Danshu (B*19*), and Qimen (Liv*14*) suggests hepatopathy and disorders of Gallbladder. During pneumonopathy, tenderness or nodules may be felt at Feichu (B*13*) or Zhongfu (L*1*). Moreover, Source Points are especially useful in detecting the existence of Visceral disease. For example, tenderness at Taichong (Liv*3*) suggests hepatopathy; tenderness at Shangjuxu (S*37*) suggests periappendicular abscess, etc.

The development of auriculo-acupuncture contributes to the establishment of a new diagnostic method. For details, please consult a monograph about ear needling.

It should be emphasized once more that all data collected through Four Diagnostic Examinations should be analysed comprehensively and checked against each other. The pseudo and the genuine, the appearance and the essence, the superficial and the origin should be differentiated carefully. None of these diagnostic method should be considered as absolutely and uniquely reliable.

CHAPTER III SYNDROME DIFFERENTIATION

In TCM, a specific syndrome consists of specific symptoms and signs grouped together according to theories entirely different from those of current medicine. For instance, the Exogenous Febrile Disease is composed of six syndromes: Taiyang, Yangming, Shaoyang, Taiyin, Shaoyin, and Jueyin.

Theories and methods for syndrome differentiation develop along with the recognition of new types of illness, the discovery of new therapeutic measures, and the accumulation of clinical experiences.

Differention of Eight Principal Syndromes is the basic guideline of all methods of syndrome differentiation, while differentiation of Visceral syndromes serves as its important and necessary supplement. Together with the method of Vital Energy, Blood, and Fluid syndrome differentiation and Meridian syndrome differentiation, they form a complex system, which is especially suitable for syndrome differentiation in miscellaneous internal disease.

As to epidemic febrile diseases, methods of Defence-Energy-Nutrient-Blood syndrome differentiation and Triple Energizer syndrome differentiation are adopted nowadays.

Section 1. Differentiation of Eight Principal Syndromes

Eight Principal Syndromes consist of Yin-Yang, Exterior-Interior, Cold-Heat, and Asthenia-Sthenia. Among them, Yin-Yang may be regarded as a guideline of the other six syndromes simultaneously. Characteristics of these syndromes should be learnt by heart.

Since symptoms and signs of diseases are complex and variable, different Principal Syndromes may be mixed up with each other, or transform from one to another.

Some ancient Chinese doctors regard Pseudo-Genuine as a basic principle also, which must be taken into account in the course of clinical practice.

I. *Exterior-Interior*

In TCM, the body shell, including the head and limbs, is regarded as Exterior; Viscera are regarded as Interior. Among Viscera, Hollow Viscera are regarded as Exterior, Parenchymatous Viscera are regarded as Interior.

1. Exterior syndrome

This is often encountered at the initial stage of an exopathic disease.

Its manifestations are as follows: aversion to cold or wind, pyrexia, headache, pantalgia, stuffy nose, dilute nasal discharge, white and thin coating of the tongue, floating pulse.

2. Interior syndrome

This may be caused by a direct invasion of exopathic evils, an indirect transformation from an exterior syndrome, or an internal damage due to overexertion, improper diets, excessive emotional changes, etc.

Symptoms and signs of interior syndrome are various and changeable, because the interior of the body consists of various internal organs, and their physiopathologic activities correlate intimately with each other. Details of interior syndrome will be discussed later in *Differentiation of Visceral Syndromes*.

3. Differentiation between exterior and interior syndrome

The crux of their differentiation lies in whether there is aversion to cold or wind, as well as the picture of the tongue and the pulse condition. Ancient doctors had pointed out, *Whenever there is a portion of aversion to cold (or wind), there is a portion of exterior syndrome.*

4. Complicated states of exterior syndrome and interior syndrome

1) Coexistence of exterior and interior syndrome

This may be caused by:

① A diffuse invasion of pathogenic evils throughout the body

② Simultaneous exopathic attack and interior damage, such as a common cold with dyspepsia

③ An interior syndrome has not been relieved while the body is attacked by exopathic evils

④ An exterior syndrome has not been relieved while it is transmitted interiorly

Under these circumstances, the pathogenesis is intricate and varied. Cold and Heat, Asthenia and Sthenia may get entangled, such as Cold Exterior with Heat Interior, Sthenic Exterior with Asthenic Interior, or vice versa.

2) Coming in of exterior syndrome and going out of Interior syndrome

① Coming in of exterior syndrome

This is generally due to: Decline of one's resistance to disease; excessive exuberance of pathogenic evils; inappropriate nursing, negligence of treatment, or erroneous treatment

For instance, there is originally an exterior syndrome with aversion to cold and pyrexia. After the disappearance of aversion to cold, there is aversion to heat, accompanied with thirst, frequent drinking of water, deep-coloured urine, reddened tongue, and yellow coating of the tongue.

② Going out of interior syndrome

This is usually due to: reinforced body resistance; appropriate nursing, proper and prompt treatment

For instance, there is an interior heat syndrome originally. Later on, skin rash occurs accompanied with perspiration, decrease of fever and dysphoria, etc.

5. Half exterior and half interior syndrome

This is characterized by alternate chills and fever, fullness of the chest and hypochondria, loss of appetite, dysphoria, nausea, bitter taste in the mouth, dry throat, dizziness, and stringy pulse. Such symptoms and signs were designated as Shaoyang syndrome in *Treatise on Febrile Diseases* by Zhang Zhongjing.

In Ming Dynasty (1642), Wu Youke discovered that there is also an half exterior and half interior syndrome in pestilence which is different from that in Exogenous Febrile Disease. It is characterized by aversion to cold at first, then ardent fever, headache, pantalgia, reddened tongue with thick powder-like coating, and rapid pulse.

II. *Cold and Heat*

Generally speaking, in addition to an attack of exogenous Cold, the exuberance of Yin or debility of Yang leads to a cold syndrome; the exuberance of Yang or depletion of Yin leads to a heat syndrome.

Cold or Heat may exist in its simple form, but their heterogenous and pseudo form are often encountered clinically. Cold should be treated with hot-natured drugs; Heat should be treated with cool-or cold-natured drugs. Therefore, the differentiation of Cold and Heat is of utmost importance.

1. Cold syndrome

Cold syndrome may be classified according to its location, exterior or interior, and its nature, asthenic or sthenic. Here, we only discuss Exterior Cold and Interior Cold.

1) Exterior Cold

This is characterized by aversion to cold, pyrexia, absence of sweat, headache, stiff nape, arthralgia, white and thin coating of the tongue, floating and tense pulse.

2) Interior Cold

This may also be regarded as Visceral Cold, and its manifestations are various due to the location of Cold where it takes place. Details of Interior Cold will be discussed later in *Differentiation of Visceral Syndromes*.

Generally, Interior Cold is characterized by intolerance of cold, cold limbs, pale complexion, pale tongue with white and moist coating, deep and slow pulse, or accompanied with soreness and coldness of the waist and knees, long-passing and clear urine, loose stool, etc.

2. Heat syndrome

This may be caused by an attack of exogenous Warm-Heat evil, or by the exuberance of Yang or depletion of Yin. It may be classified according to its location, exterior Heat or interior Heat, or according to its nature, asthenic Heat or sthenic Heat. Here, we only discuss Exterior Heat and Interior Heat.

1) Exterior Heat

This is characterized by slight aversion to wind and cold, moderate fever with or without perspiration, headache, slight thirst, white or yellow thin coating of the tongue, or red tip of the tongue, floating and rapid pulse.

2) Interior Heat

This may also be regarded as Visceral Heat, and its manifestations are various due to the location of Heat where it takes place. Details of Interior Heat will be discussed later in *Differentiation of Visceral Syndromes*.

Generally, Interior Heat is characterized by high fever, absence of chills, aversion to heat, thirst, longing for cold drinks, scanty deep-coloured urine, dry stool or constipation, reddened tongue with yellow coating, full and rapid pulse, etc.

3. Differentiation of cold syndrome and heat syndrome

This may be summarized as the following table:

	Cold	Heat
Aversion	Aversion to cold	Aversion to heat,
Desire	Desire to be warmed	desire to be cooled
Thirst	—	+
Complexion	pale	flushing
Limbs	cold	hot
Defecation	Loose stool	Dry stool and/or constipation
Urination	Clear, long-passing urine	Scanty, deep-coloured urine
Vitality	Listless	Fretful
Picture of the tongue	Pale tongue with white coating	Reddened tongue with yellow coating
Pulse condition	Slow	Rapid

Table 2. Differentiation between Cold and Heat

4. Complicated states of cold and heat syndrome

1) Concurrent Cold and Heat

① Heat in the upper part and Cold in the lower part of the body: Generally, this indicates conjunctival congestion, sore throat, toothache, headache, feverish sensation in the chest, sour and putrid vomitus, etc., accompanied with cold pain in the abdomen or the waist and knees, loose stool, clear and colourless urine, etc.

② Cold in the upper part and Heat in the lower part of the body: Generally, this indicates cold pain in the epigastric region, clear and watery vomitus, frequent hiccup, etc., accompanied with dry stool and stagnation, frequent urgency of micturition and urodynia, reddened, hot, swollen, and painful testis, etc.

③ Cold in the exterior and Heat in the interior of the body: Generally, this indicates aversion to cold, pantalgia, absence of sweat, floating and tense pulse, etc., accompanied with fretfulness, fever, thirst, constipation, etc.

④ Heat in the exterior and Cold in the interior of the body: Generally, this indicates slight aversion to wind and cold, swelling and pain of the throat, expectoration of yellow and sticky phlegm, floating pulse, etc., accompanied with cold pain in the abdomen, loose stools, diarrhea before dawn, clear and long-passing urine, white and slippery coating of the tongue, etc.

Confronted with concurrent Cold and Heat, we should discriminate which is the incidental, which is the substantial, as well as their mutual relationship.

2) Transformation of Cold and Heat

This indicates the transformation of a syndrome from Cold into Heat or from Heat into Cold; Cold and Heat do not exist at the same time.

① Transformation from Cold into Heat: This may be illustrated by the transormation of an exterior cold syndrome into an interior heat syndrome.

② Transformation from Heat into Cold: This may occur suddenly or gradually. A patient suffering from high fever may suddenly fall into a state of Yang exhaustion (cold sweat, cold limbs, pale complexion, hypothermia, etc.) due to profuse and incessant perspiration or excessive vomit or diarrhea. A hot dysentery (Wetness-Heat) may gradually change into a cold dysentery.

3) Pseudo and genuine Cold or Heat

In critical condition, there may be a state in which Cold may look like Heat, or Heat may look like Cold.

① Genuine Cold with pseudo Heat: This is generally caused by the outward escape of Yang due to the repelling action of exuberant Yin. For instance, there are fever, flushing, thirst, longing for cold drinks, restlessness, delirium, full and large pulse, which seem to be manifestations of a heat syndrome; but the patient desires to get clothes or quilts, does not take the cold drinks down when such drinks are fetched before him (her); he (she) wears a calm expression, speaks feebly, and his (her) pulse is weak. These reveal that the afore-mentioned symptoms and signs are not substantial.

② Genuine Heat with pseudo Cold: This is generally caused by the outward escape of Yin due to the repelling action of exuberant Yang. There are syncope, cold limbs, spontaneous perspiration, thready and indistinct pulse, which seem to be manifestations of a cold syndrome; but the patient is reluctant to be warmed and desires to be cooled and to drink cold water, and there may be dry throat, halitosis, oliguria with deep-coloured urine, fetid stool, and prickled tongue. These reveal that the afore-mentioned symptoms and signs are not substantial.

In order to discriminate a genuine state from a pseudo one, we must stick to the principle of *Comprehensive Analysis of the Data Collected from Four Disgnostic Examinations*. Moreover, the following aspects should be taken into account.

Generally speaking, pseudo Cold or Heat dominates exteriorly and superficially, genuine Cold or Heat dominates interiorly and deeply. Therefore, we rely on syndrome of the interior, picture of the tongue, and condition of the pulse.

III. *Asthenia and Sthenia*

Ancient Chinese doctors had pointed out, Asthenia implies the debility of Healthy Energy, Sthenia implies the exuberance of pathogenic evils. An asthenic state may change into a sthenic one, a sthenic state may change into an asthenic one, and there may be a heterogenous state of Asthenia and Sthenia. Moreover, Asthenia and Sthenia cannot deviate from Exterior, Interior, Cold, and Heat. Therefore, manifestations of Asthenia and Sthenia are intricate and varied.

1. Asthenic syndrome

This indicates a morbid condition characterized by the deficiency of Healthy Energy, lowered body resistance, and declined Visceral function; for example, slim or emaciated physique, listlessness, shortness of breath, intolerance of cold, tidal fever, hotness at palms and soles, anorexia, dyspepsia, loose stool, etc.

Asthenic manifestations of various internal organs will be discussed later. Here, characteristics of Vital Energy Asthenia, Yang Asthenia, Blood Asthenia, and Yin Asthenia are summarized and shown in the following table:

Asthenia of	Characteristics
Vital Energy	Feebleness, shortness of breath, low and timid voice, spontaneous perspiration, palpitation, anorexia, dyspepsia, indistinct or feeble pulse, even proctoptosis, hysteroptosis
Yang	Intolerance of cold, cold limbs, pallor, liability of sweating, loose stool, watery urine, pale lips, tastelessness, pale tongue with white and moist coating, weak pulse, even impotence
Blood	Pale complexion, pale lips, palpitation, numbness of extremities, pale tongue, thready and feeble pulse, even dry throat, thirst, insomnia, low fever in the afternoon
Yin	Low fever in the afternoon, flushed zygomatic region, hotness of palms and soles, night sweat, dry mouth, red lips, scanty and deep-coloured urine, red tongue with little coating, small and rapid pulse, even increased libido

Table 3. Characteristics of Vital Energy, Yang, Blood and Yin Asthenia

2. Sthenic syndrome

This indicates a morbid condition characterized by intense body reaction due to excessive pathogenic evils, or by the presence of pathologic products due to dysfunction of Viscera.

Sthenic manifestations of various internal organs will be discussed later. Generally, high fever, gruff respiratory sound, fixed stabbing pain in the hypochondria, distending pain of the abdomen with tenderness, constipation, dysentery with tenesmus, hydropsy, retention of urine, etc., and yellow, thick, greasy coating of the tongue signify a sthenic syndrome.

3. Differentiation between Asthenia and Sthenia

Features of Asthenia and Sthenia may be roughly summarized as follows:

	Asthenia	Sthenia
Course of disease	Protracted or chronic	Newly suffered or acute
Mental state	Listless	Excited
Voice	Low	Loud
Breath	Feeble	Gruff
Aching part	Longing for press	Resistant to press
Emotion	Melancholy, grief, fear, terror	Joy, anger
Tongue proper	Tender	Tough
Coating of the tongue	No or little	Thick
Pulse	Weak	Energetic

Table 4. Differentiation between Asthenia and Sthenia

4. Complicated Asthenia and Sthenia

1) Concurrent Asthenia and Sthenia

① Basically Sthenia, mixed with Asthenia: This may be illustrated by tympanites. In such patients, the abdomen is bulging and solid with varicose on its wall. Besides, there are sallow complexion, emaciation, edematous limbs, abdominal distension after meals, dim red prickled tongue with yellow and dry coating, relaxed weak pulse or deep, thready, rapid pulse. These symptoms and signs signify a sthenic syndrome caused by the stagnation of Vital Energy and Blood, which results in Spleen-Kidney Asthenia.

② Basically Asthenia, mixed with Sthenia: This may be illustrated by dysmenorrhea in anemic females. In such patients, there are emaciation, dry and withered skin and muscles, vexation, hotness at palms and soles, insomnia, anorexia, etc., and at the same time, there are oligomenorrhea or amenorrhea, dim purple tongue with ecchymosis, deep and stringy pulse. These are symptoms and signs of Blood Asthenia and Blood stagnation.

③ Upper Sthenia accompanied with lower Asthenia: This may be illustrated by patients suffering from hypertension. For example, there may be soreness and weakness of the waist and knees, nocturnal emission in the lower part of the body; and dizziness, headache, conjunctival congestion, etc., in the upper part of the body.

④ Upper Asthenia accompanied with lower Sthenia: This may be illustrated by patients suffering from anemia and dysentery. Under such circumstances, there will be dizziness, palpitation, vexation, insomnia, etc., and abdominal pain, tenesmus, bloody purulent stool, etc.

2) Genuine or pseudo Asthenia and Sthenia

① Genuine Asthenia and pseudo Sthenia: This is also called the appearance of excess in extreme deficiency. For example, in serious Blood deficiency there may be high fever, full and large pulse, as if it were a sthenic heat syndrome of Yangming. But under these circumstances, the pulse is hollow on heavy pressing, the tongue is pale or tender red and without deep yellow coating.

② Genuine Sthenia and pseudo Asthenia: This is also called the appearance of deficiency in extreme excess. For example, in exuberance of Heat, there may be cold limbs; and the more exuberant the Heat, the more cold the limbs. Under these circumstances, the pulse is deep-sited but energetic, the tongue is crimson, with or without scorched yellow coating; or there may be high fever, delirium, coma.

A sthenic syndrome should be treated by tonifying method, an asthenic syndrome should be treated by purgation or reduction. Therefore, the differentiation of genuine and pseudo Asthenia or Sthenia is of utmost importance in clinical practice, just as that of genuine and pseudo Cold or Heat.

IV. *Yin and Yang*

Yin and Yang may be regarded as a guideline of the other six principal syndromes, or as a pair of specific syndromes contrary to each other. The latter denotes syndromes caused by disorders of Genuine Yin and Genuine Yang of the body.

1. Yin and Yang as a guideline in Differentiation of Eight Principal Syndromes

According to theories of TCM, Interior, Cold, and Asthenia belong to Yin; Exterior, Heat, and Sthenia belong to Yang. Whether it is a Yin syndrome or a Yang syndrome may be judged by their characteristics.

	Yin	Yang
Inspection	Facing a dark corner, aversion to light, lying with crooked body, limbs, and closed eyes; disinclination to see people, chilly expression	Facing outwardly, lying supinely with stretched limbs and opened eyes, longing to see people, fretfulness, restlessness
Auscultation	Taciturnity, Weak breathing	Talkativeness, Gruff breathing
Interrogation	Desire to be warmed, no thirst, clear and long-passing urine, loose stool	Desire to be cooled, thirst, polydrinking of water, constipation, deep-coloured urine
Pulse feeing & palpation	Deep or slow pulse; coldness of the body and limbs, dry and withered skin	Floating or rapid pulse; hotness of the body and limbs, moist and smooth skin

Table 5. Characteristics of Yin Syndrome and Yang Syndrome

2. Syndromes of Genuine Yin and Genuine Yang

Genuine Yin is also called *Genuine Water, Primordial Yin, Kidney Yin*, etc.; Genuine Yang is also called *Genuine Fire, Primordial Yang, Kidney Yang*, etc. Thus, it is clear that Traditional Chinese doctors regard Kidney as a Vital Gate from which Congenital Yin and congenital Yang promote the vitality of every constituent part of the body, especially its

Parenchymatous Viscera.

Specific syndromes of Kidney as an internal organ will be discussed later in *Differentiation of Visceral Syndromes*.

1) Deficiency of Genuine Yin and Debility of Genuine Yang

According to viewpoints of Cheng Guopeng in *Medicine Comprehended* (1732), "If there are rapid, weak pulse, flaming up of asthenic Fire now and then, dry mouth, scorched tongue, interior heat, constipation, and adverse uprising of Vital Energy, these indicate the deficiency of Genuine Yin; if there are large, weak pulse, lassitude, pale tongue, normal taste of the mouth, cold skin and muscles, loose stool, and dyspepsia, these indicate the debility of Genuine Yang".

2) Yin exhaustion and Yang exhaustion

These are critical symptoms and signs which often occur gradually or suddenly during high fever, excessive vomit or diarrhea, profuse hemorrhagia, and/or copious perspiration.

According to viewpoints of Xu Dazhuang (Qing Dynasty), "During Yin exhaustion, there are exuberance of heat, thirst, longing for cold drinks, gruff breathing; hot skin, muscles, and limbs; full and replete pulse; the sweat is hot and salty in taste. During Yang exhaustion, there are intolerance of cold, cold skin, muscles, and limbs; no thirst, longing for hot drinks, faint breathing; indistinct, hollow, and rapid pulse; the sweat is cool, tasteless, and slightly sticky."

V. *Complicated states of Eight Principal Syndromes*

Exterior and Interior denote the localization of a morbid state; Cold and Heat denote the nature of a morbid state; Asthenia and Sthenia denote the relative dominance of Healthy Energy and pathogenic evils. Therefore, they are inseparable from each other. Various pathologic conditions may be classified as Exterior-Cold, Exterior-Heat, Exterior-Asthenia, Exterior-Sthenia; Interior-Cold, Interior-Heat, Interior-Asthenia, Interior-Sthenia; Exterior-Heat with Interior-Cold, Exterior-Cold with Interior-Heat, Exterior-Asthenia with Interior-Sthenia, Exterior-sthenia with Interior-Asthenia; Cold in both Exterior and

Interior, Heat in both Exterior and Interior, Asthenia in both Exterior and Interior, Sthenia in both Exterior and Interior.

Under these circumstances, which is the primary, which is the secondary; which is the substantial, which is the incidental; which is the genuine, which is the pseudo; as well as which is the urgent, which may be posponed, should be analysed and discriminated carefully.

ANNEX   Illustrative Medical Reports (Abridged)

1. "Yu Guozhen, male, adult; suffered from exogenous febrile disease for 6~7 days. Chilly body with conjunctival congestion; asking for water, but no desire to drink it; extraordinary restlessness; the door and window of his room are widely opened. The patient lies on the ground, tossing and turning uncomfortably. Furthermore, he begs to let him enter a well. His pulse is extremely full and large, but feeble on heavy pressing. Hence, this is a case of pseudo Exterior Heat with genuine Interior Cold, the asthenic Yang is about to escape...." (pp. 26~27. *Comments on Ancient and Modern Case Reports*, Yu Zhen, 1778).

2. "Female, adult; sudden coma; coldness all over the body; no perspiration; all six radial portions are deep-sited; has been remained in such a condition for 4 days; failed to respond to hot-natured drugs. I put a piece of water-drenched cloth on her body; within a short period, her body becomes hot. Thereafter she drinks cold water for 5~6 bowls, and still feels thirsty. When another bowl of cold water has been taken, profuse sweating occurs.... This is a case of *Extreme Heat looks like Cold.*" (p. 53, ibid.)

3. "Zhu Zhongwen, male, adult; intolerance of cold in summer, thickly clothed; taking very hot water and food constantly; vomit occurs whenever slightly warm edibles are swallowed....dI found his pulse is rapid and large, no weak condition can be felt. This is a case of *Extreme Fire looks like Water.*" (p. 115, ibid.)

4. "Han Maoyuan, male, adult; suffered from exogenous febrile disease for 8~9 days. He is unable to speak, to see, and to move; four extremities are cold; six portions of the radial artery cannot be felt. On abdominal palpation, he knits his brows and shields his abdomen from being pressed with both hands. I felt his pulse at the anterior tibial artery and found it is large and energetic. It is evident that there is stercoroma··· This is a case of genuine Sthenia with pseudo Asthenia." (p. 188, *Required Readings for Medical Professionals*, Li Zhongzi, 1637).

5. "Wu Wencai, male, adult; has suffered from exogenous febrile disease. There are dysphoria, confusion, feeling of extreme stuffiness, and frequent asking for cold

water. His pulse cannot be felt because of extraordinary restlessness. Assisted by 5～6 men, I found his pulse is incomparably full and large, and as thin as a silk thread on heavy pressing. This is a case of genuine Asthenia with pseudo Sthenia" (p. 188, ibid.)

6. "Sun - -, female, adult; has suffered from dysentery for 40 days; dryness of the mouth, pyrexia, no longing for food and drink, feeling of distension and oppression in the abdomen, undigested cereals in excrements. The illness had been diagnosed as dyspepsia of cereals due to evil Heat, and more than 30 dosages of a decoction composed of Radix Aucklandiae, Rhizoma Coptidis, Fructus Aurantii, Semen Myriaticae, Cortex Magnoliae Officinalis, etc., had been administered. No food has been taken for 5 days; death may come any minute.

I found her pulse was large, rapid, and magnanimous; there are abdominal pain, desire for being pressed, clear urine, and fluent micturition. Hence, this is a case of *Fire fails to generate Earth*; in other words, there are genuine Cold interiorly and pseudo Heat exteriorly" (pp. 278～9, ibid.)

7. "Chen - -, male, 18 years of age; early summer. Fever, headache, pantalgia for 3 days.

Cold limbs, unconsciousness, loss of hearing, pale complexion and lips, only the colour of finger-nails are red and lively; both pulse are deep-sited. Whether this is a cold or a heat syndrome needs to be ascertained. I bid his brother fetch a cup of cold water, prop up the patient, and try to let him drink. The patient quaffs in one gulp.

Therefore, this is a case of syncope caused by acute, exuberant Heat." (p. 75, *Classified Compilation of Proved Medical Reports from Well-Known Doctors in China* by He Lianchen, 1929)

8. "Liu - -, female, 50 years of age. Catching severe cold recently

At first, there are fever, aversion to cold; thirst, but the quantity of water taken is not much; black and moist coating of the tongue.

Three days later, There are hurried breath, wheezing of the air passage due to retention of phlegm, tender red complexion, unconsciousness, clammy limbs, dripping perspiration; floating, slippery, and thready pulse at both Inch; hollow pulse at both Cubit.

This is the so-called *genuine Cold in the lower part of the body and pseudo Heat in the upper part.*" (p. 76, ibid.)

9. "Li - -, female, 30 years of age. Habitual overeating of raw and cold diet, dyspepsia; debilitated constitution; attacked by Wind-Cold and Wetness in summer.

Weariness, decreasing appetite, aversion to cold, fever, dizziness and headache, thirst, dry throat, regurgitation of abundant clear saliva. Thereafter, complete loss of appetite for one month, extreme weariness and feebleness, intense thirst and frequent regurgitation of clear saliva, tidal fever, serious headache and ophthalmalgia, fullness and distension of the chest and diaphragm, lumbago, abdominal pain, dysphoria, slight yellowish urine, scorchingly dry lips, and sticky yellow coating of the tongue. Death is expected at any moment.

The pulse is found to be floating, rapid, and weak.

This is a state of genuine Cold with pseudo Heat. " (p. 78, ibid.)

Section 2. Differentiation of Visceral Syndrome

Differentiation of Visceral syndrome is aimed at finding out the specific locale and nature of the pathologic change or changes according to the theory of Outward Manifestations of Viscera, in which the method of Eight Principal Syndromes Differentiation is incorporated.

I. *Differentiation of Heart syndrome*
   1. Heart Asthenia
   1) Asthenia of Heart Energy

This is characterized by palpitation, shortness of breath (such symptoms are aggravated during physical activities), oppressed feeling in the precordial region, spontaneous perspiration, weak or irregular pulse.

Analogous symptoms and signs are often encountered in debilitated patients, or patients suffering from anemia, arrhythmia, neurasthenia, etc.

   2) Unconsolidation of Heart Energy

This is characterized by unsettledness of mind, mental aberration, amnesia, liability to be frightened, palpitation, severe palpitation, spontaneous perspiration, polyhidrosis, or onset of perspiration during slight physical movement, etc.

   3) Asthenia of Heart Yang

This may be regarded as an aggravated state of Heart Energy Asthenia. In addition to manifestations of Heart Energy Asthenia, there are cold limbs, intolerance of cold, profuse perspiration, severe palpitation, even coma, indistinct pulse.

Analogous symptoms and signs are often encountered in patients suffering from heart failure, or shock, etc.

4) Asthenia of Heart Blood

This is characterized by dizziness, pallor, palpitation, dysphoria, insomnia, and thready, weak pulse.

Analogous symptoms and signs are often encountered in patients suffering from neurasthenia, anemia, etc.

5) Asthenia of Heart Yin

This is characterized by palpitation, dysphoria, insomnia, amnesia, or even low fever in the afternoon, night sweat, dryness of the mouth, reddened tongue with little moisture, faint or rapid pulse.

Analogous symptoms and signs are often encountered in patients suffering from neurasthenia, anemia, tuberculosis, etc.

6) Sudden collapse of Heart Yang

This is characterized by sudden onset of profuse, dripping, cold perspiration; cold limbs, faint breath, cyanotic lips, even loss of consciousness, etc.

Analogous symptoms and signs are often encountered in patients suffering from cardiomyopathy, pulmonary heart disease, etc.

2. Heart Sthenia

1) Stagnation of Heart Blood

This is characterized by palpitation, pain or feeling of oppression in the precordial region, or even cyanosis of complexion, lips, and fingernails; cold clammy limbs, dim red tongue with little coating, faint or uneven pulse.

Analogous symptoms and signs are often encountered in patients suffering from myocardial infarction, etc.

2) Mental confusion due to the accumulation of Phlegm

Mental confusion, wheezing due to excessive phlegm, spitting of frothy saliva, feeling of oppression in the chest, even coma; white and greasy coating of the tongue, slippery pulse. This is often encountered in patients suffering from stroke, etc.

There is another type of such confusion due to the accumulation of

Phlegm and characterized by sudden falling, clouding of consciousness, clonic convulsion, superduction, spitting of frothy saliva, and accompanied with bleating like a sheep or grunting like a hog. This is often encountered in patients suffering from epilepsy, etc.

3) Heart disturbed by Phlegm-Fire

This is characterized by deranged mental state, incoherent talk, mania, capricious laughing or weeping, vexation, insomnia, reddened tip of the tongue with yellow and greasy coating, slippery and rapid pulse.

This is often encountered in exogenous febrile disease.

3. Heart Heat

1) Exuberance of Heart Fire

This is characterized by flushing, vexation, feeling of hotness within the chest, insomnia, severe palpitation, restlessness, incessant joyfulness and laughing, deep-coloured urine, even delirium, mania, hematemesis, or epistaxis.

2) Transmission of Heart Heat to Small Intestine

This is characterized by vexation, aphtha, oral ulceration, insomnia, etc., accompanied with scanty deep-coloured urine, ardor urinae, difficulty in micturition, hematuria, etc.

II. *Differentiation of Small Intestine syndrome*

1. Asthenia-Cold of Small Intestine

This is characterized by vague pain in the lower abdomen, desire to be pressed and warmed, borborygmus, diarrhea, frequent micturition, pale tongue with white coating, relaxed and weak pulse.

2. Sthenia-Heat of Small Intestine

This is characterized by dysphoria, oral ulceration, deep-coloured urine, ardor urinae, distension of the lower abdomen, yellow coating of the tongue, slippery and rapid pulse.

III. *Differentiation of Spleen syndrome*

1. Spleen Asthenia

1) Asthenia of Spleen Energy

This is characterized by feeling of exhaustion, anorexia or abdominal distension after meals, accompanied with dizziness, lassitude, sallow complexion, etc.

Analogous symptoms and signs are often encountered in gastrointestinal ulcer, gastroneurosis, chronic dysentery, etc.

2) Asthenia of Spleen Yang

This is characterized by cold pain in the gastric region, fullness and distension of the abdomen, hiccup, vomit, poor appetite, loose stools, or protracted diarrhea or dysentery, lassitude, oliguria, edema, emaciation, pale tongue with white coating, feeble and relaxed pulse.

Analogous symptoms and signs are often encountered in patients suffering from gastrointestinal ulcer, chronic gastroenteritis, chronic hepatitis, etc.

3) Asthenia of Spleen Yin

This is characterized by dryness of the mouth and lips, longing for drinking water, tastelessness, poor appetite, dry and stagnated stool, reddened tongue with little moisture and coating, or glossy tongue, etc.

4) Dysfunction of Spleen in transport

This is characterized by abdominal distension, anorexia, dyspepsia, increased borborygmus, diarrhea; and in chronic cases, sallow complexion, emaciation, feebleness of four limbs, or the accumulation of Fluid or Phlegm.

5) Failure of Spleen to keep Blood flowing within the vessels

This is characterized by chronic hemorrhage, such as menorrhagia, metrorrhagia and metrostaxis, epistaxis, and subcutaneous hemorrhage, etc.

2. Spleen Sthenia

Wetness-Heat in Spleen-Stomach is characterized by jaundice, fullness and distension of the epigastric abdomen, poor appetite, nausea, lassitude, scanty deep-coloured urine, yellow and greasy coating of the tongue, soft and rapid pulse.

Analogous symptoms and signs are often encountered in patients suffering from icteric hepatitis and other acute liver and gallbladder troubles.

IV. *Differentiation of Stomach syndrome*

    1. Stomach Asthenia

    1) Asthenia of Stomach Energy

This is characterized by feeling of fullness in the epigastric region, anorexia or dyspepsia, eructation, even vomit after meals, loose stool, pale lips and tongue.

Analogous symptoms and signs are often encountered in patients suffering from chronic gastritis, gastroptosis, etc.

    2) Asthenia of Stomach Yin

This is characterized by dryness of the mouth and lips, longing for drinks, pyrosis, vague pain in the stomach, poor appetite, dry and stagnated stool, scanty urine, even retching, hiccup, reddened tongue with little moiture, thready and rapid pulse.

Analogous symptoms and signs are often encountered in patients suffering from chronic gastritis, gastroneurosis, etc.

    2. Stomach Sthenia

    1) Retention of food in the stomach

This is characterized by distension and pain of the stomach, resistant to pressing; belching with putrid odour, vomit, anorexia; thick and greasy coating of the tongue, slippery pulse.

Analogous symptoms and signs are often encountered in patients suffering from dyspepsia, gastritis.

    2) Blood stasis in the stomach

This is characterized by fixed, stabbing epigastralgia, resistant to pressing; hematemesis with purplish black blood clots, or tarry stool; dim reddened tongue with ecchymosis, thready and uneven pulse.

Analogous symptoms and signs are often encountered in patients suffering from gastroduodenal ulcer, chronic gastritis, etc.

    3. Stomach Cold

This is characterized by cold gastralgia relieved by warming, watery vomitus, tastelessness, preference for hot drinks, loose stool, white and moist coating of the tongue.

4. Stomach Heat

1) Stomach Heat

This is characterized by thirst, halitosis, hyperorexia, oliguria with deep-coloured urine, constipation, etc.

2) Exuberance of Stomach Heat

This is characterized by polydipsia, longing for cold drinks, halitosis, erosion of lips, periodontitis, pyrosis, oliguria with deep-coloured urine, constipation, reddened tongue with thick and yellow coating. In epidemic febrile disease, there may be coma, delirium, restlessness, etc.

V. *Differentiation of Lung syndrome*

1. Lung Asthenia

1) Asthenia of Lung Energy

This is characterized by pale complexion, shortness of breath, low and feeble voice, aversion to wind, spontaneous perspiration, etc.

2) Asthenia of Lung Yin

This is characterized by dry cough, tidal fever, night sweat, flushing of the zygomatic region, hotness at palms and soles, dry throat and hoarse voice, dry and reddened tongue, thready and rapid pulse.

Analogous symptoms and signs are often encountered in patients suffering from pulmonary tuberculosis, chronic pharyngitis, etc.

2. Lung Sthenia

1) Attack of Wind-Cold on Lung

This is characterized by chills, stuffy nose, speaking with a twang, sneezing, profuse watery nasal discharge, thin sputum, headache, absence of perspiration, white and thin coating of the tongue, floating pulse.

2) Accumulation of Phlegm-Heat in Lung

This is characterized by fever, cough, wheezing due to the collection of phlegm in the air passage, feeling of fullness and oppression in the chest, expectoration of sticky, yellow sputum or blood-stained sputum, even dyspnea, chest and hypochondriac pain; reddened tongue with yellow and greasy coating, slippery and rapid pulse.

Analogous symptoms and signs are often encountered in patients suffering from acute bronchitis, pneumonia, etc.

3) Accumulation of Phlegm-Wetness in Lung

This is characterized by cough with copious white and thin sputum which is easily expectorated, feeling of fullness and oppression in the chest; white, and slippery or greasy coating of the tongue, soft and relaxed pulse.

Analogous symptoms and signs are often encountered in patients suffering from chronic bronchitis, bronchial asthma, etc.

4) Obstruction of Lung by Cold-Phlegm

This is characterized by intolerance of cold, cold sensation on the back, dyspnea, white and thin or frothy sputum, white coating of the tongue, slow pulse.

5) Impairment of Lung by Dryness

This is characterized by dry cough, dry nose, itching and sore throat, thirst; chest and hypochondriac pain, even bloody sputum; reddened tongue, thready and rapid pulse.

VI. *Differentiation of Large Intestine syndrome*

1. Asthenia of Large Intestine

This is characterized by proctoptosis, protracted diarrhea, undigested cereals in pale stool with little fetid odour, borborygmus, etc.

2. Asthenia-Cold of Large Intestine

This is characterized by diarrhea with loose stool, intolerance of cold, cold limbs, vague pain of the abdomen which may be relieved by warming and pressing, thin coating of the tongue, deep and thready pulse.

Analogous symptoms and signs are often encountered in patients suffering from chronic enteritis, chronic dysentery, etc.

3. Deficiency of Fluid in Large Intestine

This is characterized by dry and stagnated stool, dyschesia, accompanied with emaciation, dryness of the skin, dry throat, reddened tongue with little coating, thready pulse.

Analogous symptoms and signs are often encountered in patients suffering from senile or habitual constipation, or constipation in later stage of febrile diseases.

4. Invasion of Large Intestine by Heat

This is characterized by acute diarrhea with abdominal pain, yellow and fetid feces, burning sensation of the anus, scanty deep-coloured urine, yellow and greasy coating of the tongue, slippery and rapid pulse.

5. Heat constipation

This is characterized by constipation with abdominal distension and pain, resistant to pressing; dry and yellow coating of the tongue, deep, replete, and energetic pulse.

6. Wetness-Heat of Large Intestine

This is characterized by discharging of purulent and bloody stools, abdominal pain, tenesmus, scanty deep-coloured urine, yellow and greasy coating of the tongue, slippery and rapid pulse.

Analogous symptoms and signs are often encountered in patients suffering from dysentery, acute enteritis, etc.

7. Intestinal abscess

This generally indicates appendicitis, including its complications.

VII. *Differentiation of Kidney syndrome*

1. Unconsolidation of Kidney Energy

This is characterized by spermatorrhea, premature ejaculation, nocturia, enuresis, incontinence of urine.

Disorders of Kidney are often associated with sexual dysfunction.

2. Asthenia of Kidney Yang (or Genuine Yang)

This is characterized by intolerance of cold, cold limbs, soreness of the waist, spermatorrhea, impotence, polyuria at night, even listlessness, lumbago, chilly sensation in the spine, diarrhea before dawn, or edema; pale and corpulent tongue; deep, slow, and indistinct pulse.

3. Asthenia of Kidney Yin (or Genuine Yin)

This is characterized by lumbago, lassitude, dizziness, tinnitus, nocturnal emission, premature ejaculation, dry mouth, sore throat, flushed zygomatic region, hotness at palms and soles, tidal fever, reddened tongue with little or no coating, thready and rapid pulse.

4. Hyperactivity of Ministerial Fire

Ministerial Fire assists Monarch (or Heart) Fire in warming Viscera and maintaining their activities. It originates from Vital Gate and resides in Liver, Gallbladder, and Triple Energizer. Its hyperactivity is characterized by vertigo, headache, tinnitus, irritability, excessive dreaming during sleep, spermatorrhea, hypererosia, etc.

5. Edema due to Kidney Asthenia

This is characterized by lumbago, intolerance of cold, cold limbs, white and moist coating of the tongue, deep and thready pulse.

Analogous symptoms and signs are often encountered in patients suffering from chronic nephritis.

6. Failure of Kidney in receiving air

This is characterized by dyspnea, shortness of breath, and prolonged expiration.

VIII. *Differentiation of Urinary Bladder syndrome*

1. Asthenia-Cold of Urinary Bladder

This is characterized by intolerance of cold, cold limbs, chilly feeling in the lower abdomen, frequent micturition, enuresis, dribbling of urine, clear and light-coloured urine, white and moist coating of the tongue, thready and weak pulse.

Analogous symptoms and signs are often encountered in feeble, aged people; or in patients suffering from protracted serious illness.

2. Wetness-Heat of Urinary Bladder

This is characterized by frequent, urgent micturition, dysuria, urodynia, deep-coloured or bloody urine, fullness and distension of the lower abdomen, reddened tongue with yellow and greasy coating, rapid pulse.

Analogous symptoms and signs are often encountered in patients suffering from acute cystitis.

IX. *Differentiation of Liver syndrome*

1. Liver Asthenia

1) Asthenia of Liver Energy

This is characterized by palle complexion and lips, feebleness, tinnitus, deafness, liability to be frightened.

2) Asthenia of Liver Blood

This is characterized by sallow complexion, impaired vision, dizziness, numbness of limbs, vexation, insomnia, irregular menstruation, scanty menses, stringy and thready pulse.

Analogous symptoms and signs are often encountered in patients suffering from anemia, neurasthenia, hypomenorrhea, etc.

3) Asthenia of Liver Yin

This is characterized by dizziness, headache, blurred vision, dryness of the eye, night blindness, amenorrhea, oligomenorrhea.

Analogous symptoms and signs are often encountered in patients suffering from hypertension, neurasthenia, etc.

2. Liver Sthenia

1) Stagnation of Liver Energy

This is characterized by emotional depression, irritability, distending or wandering pain of the chest and hypochondria, feeling of oppression in the chest, distending pain of the breast, irregular menstruation, or accompanied with gastralgia, acid regurgitation, anorexia, etc.

2) Wetness-Heat of Liver Meridian

This is characterized by incessant dripping of sticky and foul discharge from the vagina, accompanied with stuffiness in the breast, dizziness, bitter taste, and dry throat.

3) Wetness-Heat in Liver and Gallbladder

This is characterized by jaundice, fever, bitter taste, pain in the hypochondrium, nausea, vomit, anorexia, aversion to fatty food, abdominal distension and pain, yellowish urine, loose stools; yellow and greasy coating of the tongue, stringy and rapid pulse.

Analogous symptoms and signs are often encountered in patients suffering from acute icterohepatitis, cholangitis, etc.

3. Liver Heat

1) Liver Heat

This is characterized by bitter taste, dry throat, vexation and feeling of fullness and oppression in the chest and hypochondria, restlessness, dizziness, conjunctival congestion, irritability; redness of the lateral side of the tongue with yellow coating, stringy and rapid pulse.

2) Liver Fire

This is characterized by headache, dizziness, conjunctival congestion, impairment of hearing, distending pain in eyeballs, irritability, restlessness, bitter taste, dysphoria, or even mania, hematemesis, hemoptysis, epistaxis; redness of the lateral side of the tongue with yellow coating; stringy, rapid, and energetic pulse.

4. Liver Cold

1) Liver Cold

This is characterized by melancholy, timidity, weariness, liability to be fatigued, cold limbs; deep, thready, and slow pulse.

2) Accumulation of Cold in Liver Meridian

This is characterized by distension, fullness, cold sensation, and pain of the lower abdomen, dragging pain in testicles, intolerance of cold, cold limbs, white and slippery coating of the tongue, deep and stringy pulse or slow pulse.

Analogous symptoms and signs are often encountered in patients suffering from disorders of testis, epididymis, hernia, etc.

5. Miscellaneous syndromes of Liver

1) Upward hyperactivity of Liver Yang

This is characterized by dizziness, headache, flushed face, blurred vision, tinnitus, bitter taste, reddened tongue, stringy and slippery or thready pulse.

Analogous symptoms and signs are often encountered in patients suffering from hypertension.

2) Adverse uprising of Liver Energy

This is characterized by dizziness, headache, flushed face, tinnitus, deafness, fullness and pain of the chest and hypochondria, belching, acid regurgitation, even hematemesis, stringy and energetic pulse.

3) Hyperactive Liver attacks Stomach

This is characterized by dizziness, feeling of oppression in the chest, hypochondriac pain, irritability, irascibility, epigastric distension and pain, anorexia, nausea, vomit, acid regurgitation; stringy pulse.

4) Upward stirring of Liver Wind

This is characterized by dizziness, vertigo, twitching of limbs, tremor, spasm, convulsion, sudden loss of consciousness, falling, deviation of the eyes and mouth, superduction, etc.

Analogous symptoms and signs are often encountered in patients suffering from serious dysfunction of the central nervous system.

X. *Differentiation of Gallbladder syndrome*

1. Asthenia of Gallbladder (Energy)

This is characterized by insomnia, vexation, panic, palpitation, liability to be frightened, apprehension, frequent heaving of sighs, etc.

Analogous symptoms and signs are often encountered in patients suffering from hysteria, neurasthenia, etc.

2. Sthenia of Gallbladder

This is characterized by feeling of fullness and oppression in the chest and epigastric region, distending pain of the hypochondrium, bitter taste, dry mouth, aching of the temporal regions, pain in the outer canthi.

3. Heat of Gallbladder

This is characterized by feeling of vexation and oppression in the chest and hypochondrium, bitter taste, dry throat, bile regurgitation, dizziness, blurred vision, deafness, alternate attacks of chills and fever, jaundice, etc.

XI. *Differentiation of Pericardium syndrome*

1. Attack of Pericardium by Heat

This is characterized by high fever, coma, delirium, or lethargy and keeping of silence, etc.

2. Obstruction of Pericardium Aperture by Phlegm

This is characterized by mental confusion, wheezing due to the retention of phlegm in the air passage, feeling of oppression in the chest, even coma; white and greasy coating of the tongue, slippery pulse.

Analogous symptoms and signs are often encountered in patients suffering from encephalitis B, epidemic encephalitis, stroke, epilepsy, etc.

XII. *Differentiation of Triple Energizer syndrome*

1. Asthenia-Cold of Triple Energizer

This indicates the Asthenia-Cold of Heart and Lung (Upper Energizer), Spleen and Stomach (Middle Energizer), and Liver and Kidney (Lower Energizer).

2. Sthenia-Heat of Triple Energizer

This indicates the Sthenia-Heat of Heart and Lung (Upper Energizer), Spleen and Stomach (Middle Energizer), and Liver and Kidney (Lower energizer).

XIII. *Complicated syndromes of Parenchymatous Viscera*

1. Breakdown of the nomal physiological coordination between Heart and Kidney

This is characterized by vexation, insomnia, dreaminess, palpitation, seminal emission, etc.

Analogous symptoms and signs are often encountered in patients suffering from neurasthenia, protracted illness, etc.

2. Asthenia of both Heart and Spleen

This is characterized by palpitation, amnesia, insomnia, dreaminess, anorexia, loose stools, abdominal distension, weariness and lassitude, sallow complexion, emaciation; pale tongue with white coating; thready, weak pulse.

Analogous symptoms and signs are often encountered in patients suffering from neurasthenia, anemia, etc.

3. Stagnation of Liver Energy and Spleen Asthenia

This is characterized by hypochondriac pain, anorexia, abdominal distension, loose stools, weariness of limbs, etc.

4. Incoordination between Liver and Spleen

This is characterized by hypochondriac distension and / or pain, eructation, anorexia, abdominal distension and pain, increased borborygmus, flatulence, loose stools, irritability, stringy and slow pulse.

5. Yin Asthenia of Liver-Kidney

This is characterized by dizziness, distending pain of the head, blurred vision, tinnitus, dry throat and mouth, soreness and weakness of the waist and knees, dry and reddened tongue, thready and feeble pulse.

6. Asthenia of both Spleen and Lung

This is characterized by pale complexion, cold limbs, poor appetite, loose stools, shortness of breath, cough, copious expectoration, emaciation, spontaneous perspiration; pale tongue with white coating, thready and weak pulse.

7. Asthenia of both Lung and Kidney

This may be classified as two types:

1) Asthenia of Lung-Kidney Energy

This is characterized by dyspnea, shortness of breath, spontaneous perspiration, polyhidrosis, soreness and weakness of the waist and knees, appearance of feeling cold, cold limbs, or cough with copious sputum.

2) Asthenia of Lung-Kidney Yin

This is characterized by dry cough, shortness of breath, dry throat, soreness and weakness of the waist and knees, hectic fever, seminal emission, night sweat, etc.

8. Yang Asthenia of both Spleen and Kidney

This is characterized by edema, glossy pale complexion, intolerance of cold, cold limbs, poor appetite, abdominal distension after meals, loose stools, soreness and weakness of the waist and limbs, weariness, scanty urine; pale tongue with thin coating, deep and weak pulse.

ANNEX Illustrative Medical Reports (Abridged)

1. "Zhang - -, female, 58 years of age.

Cough, dyspnea, inability to lie flat for 3 months

Sitting posture supported by pillows; flushed face, depressed expression, haggardness, dysphoria, halitosis; oppressive pain in the chest, difficulty in expectoration, dyspnea, insomnia, fever in the afternoon, anorexia, dry stool, deep-coloured urine; purplish red lips; purplish red tip of the tongue with yellowish white and thick coating; slippery, rapid, and energetic pulse.

Diagnosis: Protracted accumulation of Wetness in Lung; Obstruction of Lung Aperture by Phlegm-Fire" (p. 5, *Compilation of Clinical Experiences of Veteran Traditional Chinese Doctors*, 1st Collection, People's Publishing House, 1977).

2. "Ma - -, male, 57 years of age.

Vertigo (dizziness) for 3 years; tinnitus, palpitation, shortness of breath, lassitude and weariness, distension of the stomach, poor appetite, aching of the knee-cap; obese constitution, moving slowly, dysphoria, flushed face, cyanotic lips; purplish red tongue with thick and white coating whose middle part is yellow in colour; stringy, slippery, and energetic pulse.

Diagnosis: Vertigo due to the depletion of Liver-Kidney Yin and hyperactivity of Liver Yang" (p. 7, ibid.)

3. "Zhang - -, male, 40 years of age.

Palpitation for 1 year; tachypnea, shortness of breath, insomnia, amnesia, vertigo, lassitude, depressed and intranpuil expression, pale complexion with flushed zygomatic region, emaciated constitution, pale lips; pale tongue without coating; rapid and feeble pulse.

Diagnosis: Floating of Yang due to depletion of Yin; breakdown of the normal physiological coordination between Heart and Kidney" (p. 44, ibid.).

4. "Lan - -, male, 36 years of age.

Gastralgia, epigastric distension and fullness, poor appetite, dyspepsia for 7 years

Feeling of oppressive pain in the right lower abdomen with local hardness and tenderness; irregular defecation, putrid stools, vague gastralgia, distension and fullness in the stomach, poor appetite, emaciated constitution, dry and rough skin, pale complexion, depressed expression, shortness of breath; pale red tongue with white and thin coating; weak Cun pulse; stringy, slippery, and weak Bar pulse; feeble Cubit pulse.

Diagnosis: Stagnation of Liver Energy involving Spleen, resulting in its dysfunction to transport and transform, as well as dyspepsia" (p. 20, ibid.).

5. "Wang - -, male, 38 years of age.

Impotence for about 2 years; sometimes spermatorrhea, cloudy urine at the end of micturition; coldness in the lower half of the body below the waist, palpitation, shortness of breath, insomnia, amnesis, obese constitution, dim blackish complexion, listlessness, weariness, intolerance of cold, feeble and low voice, pale lips; pale tongue without coating; stringy, thready, and weak pulse; deep and slow at Cubit.

Diagnosis: Impotence due to depletion of both Yin and Yang" (p. 39, ibid.).

6. "Li - -, male, 70 years of age.

Walking with a crooked back, groaning repeatedly; anuria, distension of the lower abdomen; flushed face, dizziness, fever, vexation, red and dry lips; deep reddened tongue with thick and white coating whose middle part is yellow in colour; deep, rapid, and energetic pulse.

Diagnosis: Uroschesis due to the downward flow of Wetness-Heat into Urinary Bladder" (p. 22, ibid.).

7. "Wang Shishan treated a girl, 15 years of age.

Suffering from palpitation. She is in terror of being catched by someone and cannot find a place to hide herself. Struck with panic, the patient cannot fall asleep. She had been diagnosed as suffering from Heart disease and treated with relevant prescription, but failed to respond.

Wang felt her pulse and found all her six portions were thready, weak, and relaxed. Then he concluded that it is not a Heart disease, but a Gallbladder Asthenia. Decoctions for warming Gallbladder was administered and the patient was cured" (p. 179, *Comments on Ancient and Modern Case Reports* by Yu Zhen, 1778).

8. "Jing - -, male, over 60 years of age.

Distending and pricking pain of the stomach, burning sensation in the chest, pyrosis, dysphoria, restlessness, thirst, longing for drinks, oliguria, constipation. The patient cannot lie flat in bed supinely.

He had taken drugs sweet in taste and warm in nature, but symptoms and signs were aggravated.

Reddened tongue with white and slightly greasy coating; stringy, rapid, and energetic pulse.

Diagnosis: Pent-up Heat in Spleen-Stomach; Vital Energy stagnation and Blood stasis" (p. 21, *Proved Medical Reports from Xi Liangcheng*, 1978, People's Publishing House, Gansu Province).

9. "Zhang - -, female, 15 years of age.

Headache, chills and fever, chest pain induced by serious cough for two weeks; had been treated with prescriptions for relieving common cold, but failed to respond; recently, there are distending pain in the stomach and diarrhea with loose stools.

Dilute nasal discharge; expectorate white, frothy sputum; dry mouth but absence of thirst; gastralgia, borborygmus, decreased appetite, frequent diarrhea; white and slightly greasy coating of the tongue; stringy and tense pulse.

Diagnosis: Shaoyang attacked by exogenous evil; Asthenia-Cold of Spleen and Lung". (p. 7, ibid.)

10. "Li - -, male, 33 years of age.

Polydipsia, drinking 8 thermos bottles of water every 24 hrs for 2 years; frequent micturition, polyuria with thick suspension, slight cough, soreness and weakness of the waist and knees; emaciated constitution, listlessness, moving slowly, feeble voice, flushed zygomatic region, dry lips; reddened tongue with dry and yellowish white coating; thready, rapid, and weak pulse.

Diagnosis: Diabetes of the Kidney type; hyperactivity of Yang due to depletion of Yin" (p. 37, *Compilation of Clinical Experiences of VeteranTraditional Chinese Doctors*, 1st Collection, People's Publishing House, 1977).

Section 3. Differentiation of Syndromes of Vital Energy, Blood, and Fluid

Vital Energy (or Energy of various Viscera), Blood, and Fluid are manufactured and distributed by internal organs; they are material bases of functional activities of the human body. Some of their symptoms and signs have already been described in the preceding section.

I. *Differentiation of Vital Energy syndrome*

1. Asthenia of Vital Energy

This is characterized by glossy pale complexion, dizziness, tinnitus, palpitation, shortness of breath, inclination to sweat during physical movement, low and feeble voice, lassitude, weakness of limbs, etc.

Since Vital Energy is the "commander" of Blood, Asthenia of Vital Energy may result in hemorrhagic disorders, such as metrorrhagia, metrostaxis, hemafecia, epistaxis, etc.

2. Flatulence resulting from Vital Energy Asthenia

This is characterized by feeling of fullness and distension in the abdomen now and then, with a desire for being warmed or pressed, no tenderness on pressing; anorexia, pale complexion, pale lips, white and slippery coating of the tongue; weak, or large and hollow pulse.

3. Sinking of Spleen Energy (or Collapse of Vital Energy)

This is characterized by pale complexion, dizziness, inclination to sweat, shortness of breath, lassitude, anorexia, loose stools, heaviness and bearing-down sensation in the abdomen, frequent defecation, dripping urination, etc.

Analogous symptoms and signs are often encountered in patients suffering from visceroptosis. hysteroptosis, rectocele, chronic enteritis, etc.

4. Stagnation of Vital Energy

This is characterized by local distension or pain in the affected part.

5. Depression of Vital Energy

This is a special kind of pathologic change caused by emotional depression. It is characterized by feeling of distension in the chest, pain in the hypochondrium, anxiety, irritability, anorexia, menstrual disorder, etc.

6. Adverse uprising of Vital Energy

This often refers to morbid conditions of Liver, Lung, and Stomach. When Liver Energy uprises adversely, there will be vertigo, headache, flushed face, tinnitus, deafness, even coma, etc. When Lung Energy uprises adversely, there will be dyspnea, cough, etc. When stomach Energy uprises adversely, there will be belching, hiccup, or vomit, etc.

7. Fever caused by Vital Energy Asthenia

Generally speaking, Asthenia of Vital Energy results in Cold; but under certain circumstances, it leads to Heat. Such Heat may be characterized by fever with perspiration, shortness of breath, lassitude, thirst and desire for hot drinks, pale tongue with white coating, weak pulse. Drugs sweet in taste and warm in nature should be used to relieve this syndrome.

II. *Differentiation of Blood syndrome*

1. Blood Asthenia

This is characterized by pale complexion, pale lips, dizziness, palpitation, insomnia, numbness of extremities, thready and feeble pulse.

Generally speaking, Blood Asthenia is often accompanied with Vital Energy and/or Yang Asthenia. But under certain circumstances, Blood Asthenia may results in fever which is characterized by flushed face, thirst, vexation, insomnia, restlessness, full yet weak pulse. Such fever should be treated with drugs which enriches Blood.

2. Blood stasis

This is generally caused by the sluggish flow of Vital Energy due to its Asthenia, trauma, or the condensing action of Yin-Cold, etc. Its clinical manifestations vary with the locale and degree of Blood stasis or Blood stagnancy, such as abdominal pain, retarded menstruation, dysmenorrhea; or pricking pain in the chest, hematochezia, etc.

3. Blood Heat

This is characterized by nocturnal fever, dysphoria, insomnia, thirst but no longing for drinks, hemoptysis, epistaxis, hematuria, metrorrhagia, metrostaxis, etc., reddened or crimson tongue, thready and rapid pulse.

Blood Heat should be treated with drugs which may cool Blood.

4. Blood Cold

This is characterized by appearance of feeling cold, cold limbs, cold pain of the lower abdomen, desire to be warmed, dim purplish menses, irregular menstruation, dim pale tongue; deep, slow, uneven pulse.

III. *Complicated manifestations of Vital Energy and Blood syndrome*

1. Vital Energy stagnation and Blood stasis

This is generally due to the long-standing stagnation of Vital Energy which leads to Blood stasis. It is characterized by aggravation of local pain with tenderness, even formation of mass or slough.

2. Escape of Vital Energy resulting from hemorrhea

This is characterized by pale complexion, cold limbs, profuse sweating, thready and barely perceptible pulse, as seen in hemorrhagic shock.

3. Deficiency of both Vital Energy and Blood

This is characterized by concurrent deficiency of Vital Energy and Blood.

IV. *Differentiation of Fluid syndrome*

1. Deficiency of Fluid

This is characterized by dryness of the skin, lips, and throat, oliguria, dry stool, reddened tongue, thready and rapid pulse.

2. Excess of Fluid

1) Edema

① Yang edema: This is characterized by acute onset of edema starting from the head and face, accompanied with exterior syndrome, feeling of epigastric oppression, anorexia, nausea, then resulting in a state of Heat-Sthenia with hydropsy.

② Yin edema: This is characterized by gradual onset of edema, starting from the feet and legs, glossy pale complexion, listlessness, intolerance of cold, cold limbs, shortness of breath, anorexia, loose stools; soreness and weakness of the waist and knees, etc., In short, it is a state of Cold-Asthenia with hydropsy.

2) Retention of Fluid

This is characterized by the accumulation of Wetness as a pathologic product resulting from dysfunction of Lung, Spleen, and Kidney generally, or from disturbance of water circulation in the passage of Triple Energizer.

3) Phlegm

In a narrow sense, phlegm indicates the visible pathologic secretion from the lung or trachea. In a broad sense, Phlegm indicates a condensed sticky substance produced from pathologic changes, and in turn, it may be the cause of certain morbid manifestations, such as goiter, scrofula, clouding of consciousness in epilepsy, coma in stroke, etc.

Generally, in phlegm syndrome, there are greasy coating of the tonguue and slippery pulse.

ANNEX Illustrative Medical Reports (Abridged)

1. "Xu - -, female, adult.

Low fever at times, lassitude, drowsiness, especially in the afternoon. Had been treated with 2 dosages of diaphoretics; since then, there were incessant cough and stabbing pain at the hypochondrium.

Later, she was treated with prescriptions to clear Lung Heat and purge Fire. Thereafter, diarrhea occurs without stop.

Insomnia, no food has been taken for 10 days.

Glossy pale complexion, deadly cold hands, dispersed gleam of the eyes; pale, enlarged, and tender tongue with white and slippery coating; on light touch, her pulse is thready and weak; on deep pressing, relaxed and large.

Diagnosis: Damage of Spleen due to over-exertion; fever resulting from Asthenia of Vital Energy" (p. 28, *Concise Internal Medicine of TCM*, Nanjing College of TCM, Shanghai Science and Technology Press, 1959).

2. "A female adult.

Irascibility, vomit whenever she is angry; feeling of oppression in the chest and hypochondria, dysphoria, restlessness, abdominal pain, constipation, vomit immediately after meals for 8 days.

Feeble and indistinct pulse at all six portions.

Diagnosis: Depression of Vital Energy complicated by Phlegm-Fire; Blood deficiency and Stomach weakness" (p. 248, ibid.)

3. "Wang - -, female, 30 years of age.

Profuse vaginal bleeding with purplish black blood, thirst, longing for drinks, burning and stabbing pain of the urethra during micturition, flushed face, reddened tongue with light yellow coating; stringy and rapid pulse.

Diagnosis: Bleeding due to Blood Heat" (p. 77, *Proved Medical Reports from Xi Liangcheng*, 1978, People's Publishing House, Gansu Province).

4. "Wang - -, female, 50 years of age

Preceded menstrual cycle for 7-8 days with a menstrual period of 7-8 days in recent 6 months

This time, the menstruation lasts over 50 days; profuse, dripping menses, dilute and pale red in colour, mixed with tissues like well-cooked meat; dizziness, soreness of the waist and feebleness of legs; sallow complexion, pale red lips; pale red tongue; stringy and unevenpulse.

Diagnosis: Vital Energy Asthenia and Spleen debility; escape of blood from Vessels and Meridians" (p. 81, ibid.)

5. "Liu - -, female, over 30 years of age

Attacked by wind in summer, edema all over the body, her eyelids cannot be opened, serious distension in the abdomen, absence of perspiration, hot sensation in the epigastrium, dry stool, oliguria with deep-coloured urine; rapid pulse, stringy and hard on the left side, slippery and replete on the right side.

Diagnosis: Wind edema; depressed Heat in Liver-Gallbladder; Stomach Heat" (p. 736, *Records of Traditional Chinese and Western Medicine in Combination* by Zhang Xichun, 1918—1934).

6. "Zhang - -, male, 15 years of age

Sudden faint, loss of consciousness, superduction, slobbering along the corner of the mouth, clonic convulsion, even trismus with his tongue masticated, urinary and fecal incontinence. Such attack occurs at indefinite intervals since 5 years of age and lasts from 3~5 min. to half an hour. After the attack, he lives a normal life.

Normal coating of the tongue; stringy and slippery pulse.

Diagnosis: Epilepsy; accumulated Phlegm produces Heat, occurrence of Wind and case of extreme Heat" (p. 50, *Proved Medical Reports from Xi Liangcheng*, 1978, People's Publishing House, Gansu province).

7. "Yu Hengde had treated an obese female, 57 years of age; Sudden falling and loss of consciousness, rigidity of the body, trismus, loud wheezing due to excessive phlegm accumulated in the air passage; inability to drink water or soup. Floating, large, stringy, and slippery pulse at all six portions.

After an emetic and a little Moschus had been administered through her nasal aperture, the patient vomited a large quantity of phlegm and regained her consciousness. Thereafter, hemiplegia occurred.

Diagnosis: Wind stroke" (p. 71, *Concise Internal Medicine of TCM*, 1959, Nanjing College of TCM, Shanghai Science and Technology Press).

Section 4. Differentiation of Meridian Syndrome

Theories of Meridians and Collaterals are important component parts of Traditional Chinese Medicine. Through Meridians and Collaterals, Vital Energy and Blood circulate, and internal organs are connected with one another, including limbs, joints, superficial organs and tissues all over the body.

According to theories of Meridians and Collaterals, acupoints are closely related to corresponding internal organs. Needling of these acupoints may treat disorders of internal organs, and pathologic changes may also be reflected at these acupoints, especially the appearance of tenderness, nodules, or the change of skin colour.

Now, along with the development of combination of Traditional Chinese and Western Medicine, cutaneous electrical resistance of body acupoints and otopoints has been measured and found to be useful in making a diagnosis.

For details of Meridian syndrome differentiation, we may refer to a text-book of Traditional Chinese Acupuncture or related monographs.

Section 5. Differentiation of Exogenous Febrile Disease According to the Theory of Six Meridians

The method of syndrome differentiation of Exogenous Febrile Disease according to the theory of Six Meridians is incarnated in *Treatise on Febrile Disease* (Zhang Zhongjing, Han Dynasty) for the first time. Following *The Yellow Emperor's Canon of Internal Medicine*, it laid the foundation of TCM in both syndrome differentiation and therapy selection, and profoundly influenced the development of descendant TCM.

Six Meridians consist of three Yang (Taiyang, Yangming, Shaoyang) and three Yin (Taiyin, Shaoyin, Jueyin). Pathologic changes of three Yang are generally related to the exterior of the body and the six Hollow Viscera; while three Yin are generally related to the interior of the body and the five Parenchymatous Viscera. Their syndromes are recommended briefly as follows.

I. *Taiyang syndrome*

Taiyang syndrome is characterized by floating pulse, headache, stiff nape, and aversion to cold. When Taiyang syndrome is accompanied with pyrexia, sweating, aversion to wind, and relaxed pulse, it is called a Wind-stroke. When Taiyang syndrome is accompanied with pyrexia or without pyrexia, but certainly there is aversion to cold, as well as pantalgia, retching, and tense pulse at the same time, it is called an attack of Cold.

II. *Yangming syndrome*

Yangming syndrome is characterized by high fever, profuse sweating, extreme thirst, and full and large pulse. When Yangming syndrome is accompanied with aversion to heat instead of aversion to cold, it is called a Meridian syndrome of Yangming. When Yangming syndrome is accompanied with tidal fever, abdominal pain and tenderness, constipation, delirium, deep and replete pulse, it is called a

Hollow Visceral syndrome of Yangming.

III. *Shaoyang syndrome*

This is characterized by alternate fever and chills, fullness of the chest and hypochondrium, loss of appetite, vexation, nausea and / or vomit, bitter taste in the mouth, dry throat, dizziness, and stringy pulse. When there are fullness in the chest and hypochondrium, alternate fever and chills, vexation, and hypochondriac pain, it is called a Meridian syndrome of Shaoyang. When there are bitter taste in the mouth, dry throat, dizziness, feeling of oppression in the chest, and vomit, it is called a Hollow Visceral syndrome of Shaoyang.

IV. *Taiyin syndrome*

This is characterized by fullness of the abdomen, vomit, inability to take meals, diarrhea, abdominal pain, relaxed and weak pulse, while there are no pyrexia and no thirst.

V. *Shaoyin syndrome*

This is characterized by thready and indistinct pulse, desire to sleep, intolerance of cold, cold limbs, listlessness, lienteric diarrhea; or characterized by vexation, insomnia, dry mouth, reddened tongue, thready and rapid pulse.

VI. *Jueyin syndrome*

This is characterized by clammy limbs, thirst, epigastric pain with burning sensation, retching, hunger but no desire for eating, even vomiting of ascarides.

These six syndromes may occur singly or they may combine with each other; furthermore, they may be transmitted from one to another.

Section 6. Differentiation of Syndromes of Epidemic Febrile Disease

I. *Theory of Defence–Energy–Nutrient–Blood Systems*

Following Zhang Zhongjing, descendant Chinese doctors had accumulated further experience in the recognition and treatment of epidemic febrile disease. In line with theories of The Yellow Emperor's Canon of Internal Medicine, they proposed that the general course or development of such diseases may be classified as four stages and four different prescriptions had been designed which are proved to be effective.

1. Defence or the initial stage

In this stage, Defence System is attacked by epidemic febrile pathogen, and its disorder is manifestated by fever, slight aversion to wind or cold, headache, pantalgia, absence of perspiration or slight perspiration, stuffy nose, cough, slight thirst, white and thin coating of the tongue, floating and rapid pulse.

2. Energy stage

This is characterized by symptoms and signs of Energy System, such as high fever, no aversion to cold but aversion to heat, perspiration, thirst, flushing face, gruff breathing, scanty deep-coloured urine, constipation; yellow or yellow and dry coating of the tongue, full and large or slippery and rapid pulse. These may be accompanied by tidal fever, delirium, cough with yellow sputum, fullness and pain of the abdomen, or fecal impaction with watery discharge.

3. Nutrient stage

Symptoms and signs of Nutrient System are characterized by high fever which is aggravated at night, dysphoria, insomnia, or delirium, unconsciousness, but absence of thirst; indistinct skin rashes, crimson tongue with yellow and dry or grey and dry coating, thready and rapid pulse.

4. Blood System

Symptoms and signs of Blood System are characterized by high fever which is aggravated at night, dysphoria and restlessness, evident skin rashes in deep purple colour, dim purple or deep crimson tongue, thready and rapid pulse; even unconsciousness, delirium, convulsion, twitching, hematemesis, epistaxis, hematochezia. This indicates the critical stage of an epidemic febrile disease.

II. *Theory of Triple Energizer*

This is a complementary method to that of Defence-Energy-Nutrient-Blood System. It takes Upper, Middle, and Lower Energizer as the three stage of the development of epidemic febrile disease.

1. Syndrome of Upper Energizer

This indicates syndromes of Taiyin Meridian of the Hand and those of Pericardium Meridian of the Hand, which occur at the initial stage. It is characterized by fever, aversion to cold, spontaneous perspiration, headache, thirst or absence of thirst, cough, as well as unconsciousness, delirium, dysphoria, restlessness, even cold limbs, curling and stiffness of the tongue; reddened or crimson tongue, rapid pulse.

2. Syndrome of Middle Energizer

This indicates syndromes of Yangming Meridian of the Foot and those of Taiyin Meridian of the Foot. It is characterized by fever, no aversion to cold but aversion to heat, profuse perspiration, polydipsia, drinking in large draughts, or tidal fever, delirium, fullness of the abdomen with tenderness, abdominal pain around the navel, constipation; as well as recessive fever, heaviness of the body and pantalgia, feeling of oppression in the chest, nausea, fullness at the epigastric region, dyschesia or loose stools, greasy coating of the tongue, relaxed pulse.

3. Syndrome of Lower Energizer

This indicates syndromes of Shaoyin Meridian of the Foot and those of Jueyin Meridian of the Foot. It is characterized by hotness of the body, especially at palms and soles, dryness of the mouth and tongue but no longing to take much water, vexation, restlessness, insomnia, as well as cold limbs due to extreme pyrexia, pyrosis, involuntary movement of limbs, clonic convulsion. This signifies the critical stage of epidemic febrile disease.

The concept of Triple Energizer is also applicable to afebrile miscellaneous internal disease where they denote symptoms and signs of Heart-Lung, Spleen-Stomach, and Liver-Kidney respectively.

III. *Identification of Epidemic Febrile Diseases*

Epidemic febrile diseases have been identified as Wind-Warm, Spring-Warm, Wetness-Warm, Summer Fever, Autumn-Dryness, Winter-Warm, pestilence, and pyrexial malaria, etc. , according to TCM. Some of them develop in the order of Defence-Energy-Nutrient-Blood cited above, some may start from Energy, Nutrient, or Blood System directly, or switch from Defence to Nutrient or Blood directly; and there may be complicated states, such as Intense Heat in Both Energy and Blood System, Intense Heat in both Energy and Nutrient System, etc. Details of the differentiation and treatment of these epidemic febrile diseases may be found in related monographs.

ANNEX Illustrative Medical Reports (Abridged)

1 "Wang Ruiting, male, 38 years of age

Under intense heat of summer, entertained at a grand banquet, drinking revelledly and taking much fatty foods. After returning home late at night, he felt very thirsty and ate a raw radish. At dawn, there were hypochondriac pain on the right side, fever, and aversion to wind.

Headache, hotness of the body, spontaneous perspiration, aversion to wind and cold, hypochondriac pain at both sides, longing for cold drinks, vexation, serious cough, thick and sticky sputum; yellow, moist, and greasy coating on the right side of the tongue, rapid pulse.

Diagnosis: Attack of Wind-Warm on Taiyin, complicated by food retention". (p. 21, Classified Compilation of Proved Medical Reports from Well-known Doctors in China, He Lianchen, 1929)

2. "Gu - -, male, over 10 years of age

Affected by prevalent epidemic evil for 7 days

Chills and fever, absence of perspiration, swelling and pain of the throat, trismus;

close, numerous, indistinct eruption; even somniloquy like delirium; yellow, thin, and greasy coating of the tongue; depressed, rapid pulse.

Diagnosis: Epidemic throat disease; miss of relieving Exterior at the beginning; the epidemic evil is about to sink into the interior of the body". (p. 292, ibid.)

3. "Gao - -, female, 13 years of age

Headache, fever, and listless yesterday; headache aggravated yesterday evening accompanied with chills, feebleness, and general malaise; projectile vomiting for three times today morning

Slightly cyanotic complexion, haziness, extreme dysphoria, restlessness, loud screaming, or lethargy, delirium, tic of fingers; stiff neck, cool hands, hotness of the body, hemorrhagic spots on the chest wall, constipation for three days, incontinence of urine; crimson tongue with scorching yellow coating, scanty saliva in the mouth; stringy and rapid pulse.

Diagnosis: Pericardium attacked by Warm evil; intense Heat in both Energy and Blood Systems". (p. 173, *Proved Medical Reports from Xi Liangcheng*, 1978, People's Publishing House, Gansu Province)

4. "Lou - -, male, 5 years of age

Affected by prevalent epidemic evils

At first, there are aversion to cold, ardent fever, sneeze, nasal discharge, flushed cheeks, conjunctival congestion, cough, dyspnea; thereafter steaming internal heat, appearance of measles and purplish red maculae, dysphoria, restlessness, fullness of the abdomen, constipation; glossy purplish and bright red tongue; full, rapid, and energetic pulse.

Diagnosis: Measles complicated with maculae; Lung and Stomach attacked by epidemic evils." (p. 898, *Classified Compilation of Proved Medical Reports from Well-known Doctors in China*, He Lianchen, 1929)

5. "Xu Fusheng, male, 34 years of age; at the end of summer

Initially, there are aversion to cold, absence of perspiration; headache, heaviness of the body, fretfulness, aching of limbs, feeling of fullness in the chest and diaphragm, thirst but no longing for drinks, chills and fever in the afternoon, uneasy defecation with loose stool, scanty deep-coloured urine; thick, white, greasy and grey, slippery coating of the tongue; deep, thready, and relaxed pulse on the right side; stringy and tense pulse on the left side.

Diagnosis: Exterior attacked by Wetness; pathogenic evil lingers in Energy System and transforms into Heat; furthermore, being hit and hampered by Wind-Cold, the insidious evil cannot exhibit itself smoothly. This is a case of Wetness-Warm complicated with Cold." (p. 164, ibid.)

6. "Guo - -, male, 23 years of age

Sudden swelling and pain of the throat, dyspnea, alalia, thirst, hotness of the skin, aching of the head and nape, vexation, delirium, deep-coloured urine, uneven micturition, dry and stagnated stool; yellow coating of the tongue; deep, thready, and rapid pulse.

Diagnosis: Seasonal pestilence caused by Heat evil." (p. 276, *Classified Compilation of Proved Medical Reports from Well-known Doctors in China*, He Lianchen, 1929)

7. "Liu - -, female, 20 years of age

Soreness and weakness of four limbs, dizziness, serious conjunctival congestion, fullness of the chest, dyspnea, coma, delirium, even clonic convulsion, superduction, trismus; turbid coating of the whole tongue; full, large, rapid, and energetic pulse.

Diagnosis: Pestilent Winter-Warm." (p. 282, ibid.)

8. "Sun Yunshan, male, 31 years of age; summer

Edema of the face, numbness of limbs, aversion to cold, pyrexia, stiff spine, absence of perspiration, thirst, desire for tea, abdominal distress, serious aching at sacrum, indistinct skin eruption; light yellow coating at the root of the tongue with little saliva; floating and rapid pulse.

Diagnosis: Epidemic febrile disease with eruptions due to the accumulation of Heat in Yangming." (p. 271, ibid.)

9. "Liang - -, female, 25 years of age

Initially, there are aversion to cold, fever, headache, stiff nape, distending pain of the spine and waist, weariness of limbs, and thirst. After 7~8 hrs., the patient falls when she tries to stand up. Then, occur unconsciousness, trismus; limbs chill up to elbows and knees, burning hotness of the epigastrium, gruff breathing, dyspnea, dry and shrunken lips, dry teeth, conjunctival congestion, blue face. She remains in such a condition for about 24 hrs. Purple tongue with white and greasy coating; deep-sited pulse.

Diagnosis: Inward sinking of epidemic evil; "The deeper the evil Heat, the colder the limbs." (p. 272, ibid.)

10. "Guo -, male, 57 years of age

Suffered from common cold 2 weeks ago, fever, accompanied with heaviness of the head and headache, pantalgia, cough, dilute nasal discharge, sticky expectoration, dyspnea, feeling of oppression in the chest, poor appetite, bitter taste in the mouth, dry throat, slight thirst but longing for hot drink, pyrexia aggravated especially at midnight.

Dry and scorchingly hot skin, sudamina crystallina all over the chest and abdomen, dry, dim, and lustreless; white and greasy lingual coating whose middle part is yellowish black; floating and rapid pulse.

Diagnosis: Fever due to Wetness-Warm; exogenous evil lures endogenous Wetness and they join forces together." (p. 152, *Proved Medical Reports from m Xi Liangcheng*, 1978, People's Publishing House, Gansu Province).

REFERENCES

1. Yellow Emperor: *Canon of Internal Medicine*
2. Zhang Zhongjing: *Treatise on Febrile Diseases*
3. Wang Shuhe: *The Pulse Classics*
4. Chen Yan: *A Treatise on the Three Categories of Pathogenic Factors of Diseases*
5. Zhang Jiebin: *Complete Works of Zhang Jingyue* ((Ming Dynasty)
6. Li Zhongzi: *Required Readings for Medical Professionals* (ibid.)
7. Wu Youke: *Treatise on Acute Epidemic Febrile Diseases*. (ibid.)
8. Wu Tang: *Detailed Analysis of Epidemic Febrile Diseases* (Qing Dynasty)
9. Lei Feng: *On Seasonal Diseases* (ibid.)
10. Lin Peiqin: *Classified Treatment* (ibid.)
11. Zhang Xichun: *Records of Traditional Chinese and Western Medicine in Combination*, Revised edition, 1957, People's Publishing House.
11. Nanjing College of TCM: *An Outline of TCM*, 1958, People's Medical Publishing House.
12. Jiangsu TCM School: *Diagnostics of TCM*, 1958, Shanghai Medical Publishing House.
13. Yu Zhen: *Comments on Ancient and Modern Case Reporrts*, Reprined, 1959, Shanghai Science and Technology Press.
14. He Lianchen: *Classified Compilation of Proved Medical Reports from Well-known Doctors in China* Reprinted, 1959, Shanghai Science and Technology Press.
15. Nanjing College of TCM: *Concise Internal Medicine of TCM*, 1959, Shanghai Science and Technology Press.
16. Academy of TCM &. Guangdong College of TCM: *A Selection of TCM Terms Annotated*, 1973, People's Medical Publishing House.
17. People's Medical Publishing House: *Compilation of Clinical Experiences of Veteran Traditional Chinese Doctors*, 1st Collection, 1977.
18. Gansu Provincial Hospital of TCM: *Proved Medical Reports from Xi Liangcheng*, 1978, People's Publishing House, Gansu Province.

中 医 诊 断 学

邵念方　编著

王齐亮　翻译、审校

*

中国山东科学技术出版社出版
（山东省济南市玉函路）
中国山东新华印刷厂潍坊厂印刷
（山东省潍坊市工农路 99 号）
中国国际图书贸易总公司发行
（中国北京车公庄西路 21 号）
北京邮政信箱第 399 号　邮政编码 100044
1990 年（16 开）第 1 版第 1 次印刷
ISBN 7—5331—0519—2/R・139
（02500）

14—E—2458D